The
MICROBIOME
Cookbook

The
MICROBIOME
Cookbook

150 Delicious Recipes to Nourish Your
Microbiome and Restore Your Gut Health

Pamela Ellgen

Published in the United States by:
Ulysses Press
P.O. Box 3440
Berkeley, CA 94703
www.ulyssespress.com

ISBN13: 978-1-61243-597-8
Library of Congress Control Number: 2016934496

Printed in Canada by Marquis Book Publishing

10 9 8 7 6 5 4 3 2

Acquisitions editor: Casie Vogel
Managing editor: Claire Chun
Project editor: Renee Rutledge
Editor: Lauren Harrison
Proofreader: Renee Rutledge
Front cover design: what!design @ whatweb.com
Interior design/layout: what!design @ whatweb.com
Cover artwork: © stockcreations/shutterstock.com
Interior artwork: © Nikiparonak/shutterstock.com

CONTENTS

INTRODUCTION

The gastrointestinal microbiota comprises hundreds of trillions of bacteria, viruses, and fungal organisms that inhabit your intestines and live symbiotically with you. Your diet and lifestyle directly influence the health of this community, promoting either diversity, balance, and health or pathology, imbalance, and disease.

A healthy microbiome facilitates digestion, neutralizes toxins, quells inflammation, supports immunity, and improves metabolism. When the microbiome is disrupted, those functions suffer and a cascade of complications may ensue, including allergies and food sensitivities, mental health problems, weight gain, irritable bowel syndrome, and autoimmune diseases.

The Microbiome Cookbook provides you with the information and recipes to support a flourishing, healthy gut population, as well as strategies and recipes for repairing a damaged gut.

Part One of the book covers the basics of the microbiota, the organisms in your gut. It explains the importance of these organisms to your overall health and digestive function. It also covers the various lifestyle factors that affect the health of the microbiome, specifically the foods that should and should not be eaten and how they should be prepared.

Part Two of the book presents more than 100 recipes to support a healthy, diverse gut microbiome. The recipes are easy to prepare and utilize fresh, whole foods. All recipes are naturally free from gluten, refined sugar, and artificial or processed ingredients. Recipes include prebiotic foods to feed healthy bacteria and live bacterial cultures from fermented foods, including homemade yogurt, kombucha, and sauerkraut.

Part Three of the book is for people repairing a damaged gut and presents 45 additional recipes developed specifically for those suffering from irritable bowel syndrome, Crohn's disease, ulcerative colitis, celiac disease, small intestinal bacterial overgrowth, and other inflammatory conditions. The recipes in this section are paleo and as such are free from grains, legumes, dairy, industrial oils, and refined sugar. They incorporate many of the underlying principles of the Gut and Psychology Syndrome (GAPS) diet, Specific Carbohydrate Diet (SPC), and Low-FODMAP diet. Cooking methods are designed to provide easily digestible, nourishing foods that pass through the small intestine and colon without feeding pathological bacteria or further damaging the lining of the gut.

The Microbiome Cookbook provides the information and recipes you need to build and restore healthy gut flora. You'll be delighted to discover that the foods that do this are absolutely delicious and support your overall health goals as well!

THE BASICS OF MICROBIOTIA

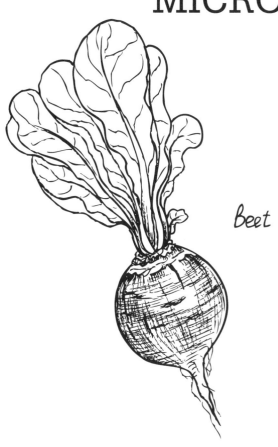

Beet

GO WITH YOUR GUT

How do you title a cookbook devoted to the indelicate topic of organisms living in your small intestine and colon? It's not exactly dinnertime conversation. But, perhaps, it should be, or at the very least, it should inform your perspective on what to eat for dinner.

The bacterial cells, viruses, and fungal organisms living in your intestinal tract outnumber human cells at least tenfold, leading some to argue that you're more bacteria than you are human. These organisms are responsible for numerous essential functions, including:

- breaking down complex carbohydrates
- producing short-chain fatty acids
- assimilating vitamins and minerals
- controlling energy assimilation
- regulating metabolism
- moderating the immune system
- maintaining mucosal barrier
- curbing inflammation
- removing toxins
- ensuring efficient elimination

In the book *Bugs, Bowels, and Behavior*, registered dietitian Geri Brewster says what we eat has a significant impact on our gut microbiota. And the rigors of a modern lifestyle, particularly stress and poor nutrition, aren't doing us any favors. "Dietary factors can shape the gut environment for the proliferation of both beneficial and pathogenic bacteria," he says.

FOOD FOR YOUR MICROBIOME

Like any organism, a healthy, diverse gut population requires sustenance. Nutrition that supports healthy microbiota includes prebiotic foods with fermentable fibers to feed the healthy bacteria, probiotic foods that are already teeming with good bacteria, and healing foods that nourish the gut lining.

PREBIOTICS

Prebiotics are food for your gut bacteria. You don't digest them yourself; your gut microbes do. Prebiotics come in the form of soluble fiber, including inulin, oligofructose, fructooligosaccharides, galacto-oligosaccharides, and other oligosaccharides. According to Mark Sisson, nutrition researcher and author of *The Primal Blueprint*, "Without fermentable fibers, our gut bacteria just aren't getting the food they need to maintain the population—let alone grow it."

Prebiotics have innumerable benefits, many of which scientific research is just beginning to uncover, including increasing good bacteria, improving mineral absorption, improving blood sugar levels, and increasing production of beneficial short-chain fatty acids. Some of the foods with the greatest concentrations of prebiotics include the following:

VEGETABLES

Cruciferous vegetables, such as cauliflower, cabbage, bok choy, broccoli, and brussels sprouts are a rich source of prebiotics as well as glucosinolates, which have anti-inflammatory and anticancer properties. Jerusalem artichokes, also called sunchokes, have a mild artichoke-like flavor and are rich in inulin—so much so that a little goes a long way. Vegetables in the allium family, including onions, shallots, leeks, and garlic, are another rich source of prebiotics. Some research indicates that garlic may exhibit an antimicrobial effect on pathological bacteria without harming healthy gut microbes.

Leafy greens, especially dandelion greens, chicory, mustard greens, chard, kale, and collard greens, also offer a generous dose of prebiotics.

Other rich sources of prebiotics among vegetables include asparagus, beets, fennel, green peas, jicama, snow peas, and sweet corn.

STARCHES

Polenta, beans, chickpeas, lentils, and other legumes offer fermentable fiber and may have positive effects on the microbiome by increasing the release of short-chain fatty acids and improving vitamin absorption. When cooked and cooled, white potatoes are an excellent source of resistant starch, which passes through the small intestine undisturbed to ferment in the colon. Cooked and cooled legumes and white rice, green bananas, plantains, yams, and sweet potatoes also offer rich sources of resistant starch. Resistant starches should be introduced gradually into the diet to avoid digestive discomfort. They may not be tolerable to those with irritable bowel syndrome, so carefully evaluate your tolerance before heaping your plate with resistant starch.

NUTS

Almonds, cashews, and pistachios are particularly rich sources of prebiotics. A study published in the journal *Anaerobe* in 2014 found that almonds and almond skins increase production of healthy gut bacteria and repress production of pathological bacteria. Pistachios may be even better, according to another study, published in the *British Journal of Nutrition,* that compared the two nuts. Pistachios also offer a limited amount of resistant starch.

FRUIT

All fruits offer prebiotics, but some are loaded with it. Some of the best options include blueberries, pomegranate, nectarines, watermelon, mango, bananas, cherries, and dried fruit. Through their effects on the microbiota, blueberries enhance immunity and may destroy pathological bacteria. Bananas have a stabilizing effect on the gut ecosystem and are anti-inflammatory.

PROBIOTICS

In today's triple-washed, conventional farming, antibacterial-everything culture, probiotics are more important than ever. While prebiotic foods encourage fermentation to happen *inside* your gastrointestinal tract, probiotic foods supply active bacterial cultures as a result of fermentation that happens *outside* the gut. Yogurt is the most well-known probiotic in Western culture, but humans have been fermenting food for millennia, and the options for delicious fermented foods are diverse. Some excellent sources of probiotics include the following:

CULTURED DAIRY

Dairy products fermented with lactic acid are more digestible; the lactic acid digests the milk sugar that causes many people digestive discomfort. Cultured dairy products include yogurt, buttermilk, crème fraîche, some cheeses, and many other regional specialties around the world. For people who cannot consume dairy products, non-dairy yogurt can also be made using almond or coconut milk.

FERMENTED SOY

Fermenting soy products not only introduces beneficial bacteria but also improves the digestibility of the legume. Some of the most widely consumed fermented soy products include tempeh, miso, soy sauce, and fermented bean curd. Tempeh in particular has been shown to improve nutrient absorption and inhibit pathological bacterial overgrowth.

FERMENTED BEVERAGES

Kefir is technically a dairy-based beverage and is made with kefir grains and dairy. Kombucha is a lightly sweetened, effervescent, fermented tea drink. Kvass is a fermented beverage that is slightly effervescent and is popular in Eastern Europe and Russia.

FERMENTED VEGETABLES

You can ferment nearly any vegetable. Some of the most popular versions include sauerkraut and kimchi. Entire books are devoted to the subject of fermented foods and offer a delicious array of fermented vegetable recipes.

HEALING FOODS

In addition to prebiotics and probiotics, some foods are particularly healing to the gastrointestinal tract. These include bone broth, gelatin, omega-3 fats, and monounsaturated fats such as olive oil. Although it does contain a significant amount of saturated fat, coconut oil has antifungal and antiviral properties, and contains lauric, capric, and caprylic acids, which combat candida; coconut oil should be added slowly to your diet because it can cause digestive distress if consumed in excess. Grass-fed organic butter also contains the antimicrobial fatty acid butyric acid and has antifungal properties.

Additionally, some foods have natural antimicrobial properties that may inhibit pathological bacterial overgrowth in the gut. These include basil, cilantro, caraway, chamomile, cinnamon, chile peppers, paprika, cranberry, garlic, grapefruit zest, green tea, hemp, nutmeg, olive oil, orange peel, papaya, peppermint, rosemary, savory, tarragon, thyme, and turmeric.

SIMPLE STEPS
FOR HEALTHY DIGESTION

1: Chew food thoroughly. Chewing mixes the food with digestive enzymes in saliva and stimulates further production of enzymes in the stomach. It also relaxes the lower stomach for improved digestion. Improperly chewed foods that pass through the stomach into the small intestine feed pathological bacteria.

2: Limit beverages at meal time. Liquids dilute and even denature salivary and stomach enzymes. If you must drink something, choose water without ice.

3: Stress less. Chronic stress can alter gut motility, mucosal secretion and mucosal blood flow, visceral sensitivity, and the composition of the microbiota. Over time it can lead to gastroesophageal reflux disease, peptic ulcers, irritable bowel disease, inflammatory bowel disease, and food allergies, according to research published in the *Journal of Physiology and Pharmacology*.

DON'T FEED THE BUGS

Nourishing a healthy microbiome also involves carefully evaluating and eliminating the substances that may damage healthy gut microbes and those that feed pathological bacteria, yeast, and fungal overgrowth. Here are some of the primary foods and drugs that can harm the microbiome:

SUGAR AND ARTIFICIAL SWEETENERS

Consuming sugar in any of its forms, especially refined sugar and high-fructose corn syrup, encourages bacterial overgrowth. Artificial sweeteners such as aspartame, sucralose, and saccharin may be even worse. They can alter the gut microbiota in susceptible individuals and contribute to glucose intolerance, which can lead to weight gain, obesity, and type 2 diabetes. Sugar alcohols are an artificial sweetener ending in the suffix -ol (xylitol, mannitol, sorbitol, etc.). They are not broken down and absorbed as energy in the small intestine, and can cause significant digestive discomfort, especially when consumed in excess.

REFINED CARBOHYDRATES

A diet that includes plenty of refined grains and starches feeds the pathological bacteria, yeast, and fungi a steady diet of glucose. The starches in these refined flours (yes, even the gluten-free versions— no, *especially* the gluten-free versions) begin converting into glucose the moment they pass your lips. Research published in the *Journal of Diabetes, Metabolic Syndrome, and Obesity* found that refined flours, sugars, and processed foods "produce an inflammatory microbiota via the upper gastrointestinal tract, with fat able to effect a 'double hit' by increasing systemic absorption of lipopolysaccharide." That not only contributes to gut dysbiosis (bacterial imbalance), but also to an increase in the net energy your body receives from the foods you eat, an essential factor in overweight and obesity.

The composition of gut microbes differs between lean and obese individuals. Most notably, the microbes called "Firmicutes" are found in greater concentrations in obese individuals and cause greater energy extraction from carbohydrates. That means that you could consume the exact same number of calories as someone with fewer Firmicutes and actually obtain *more* energy from those calories. Yikes! The good news is that the microbiota responds rapidly to changes in the diet, even in as few as a couple days. An article published in the *American Journal of Gastroenterology Supplements* in 2012 concluded, "Given the potential role of the intestinal microbiota in metabolic disorders, it is reasonable to hypothesize that restoration or supplementation of certain microbial populations may have a beneficial effect."

WHEAT AND DAIRY

Wheat and dairy alter the gut microbiota and gastrointestinal tract not only in those with celiac disease and allergies to these foods, but also among people lacking enzymes for breaking down certain carbohydrates (e.g., lactose) and those with intestinal permeability, which allows gluten and casein proteins to escape the gut and cause an immune response, systemic inflammation, and potentially trigger an autoimmune disease.

Celiac disease is an autoimmune disorder in which gluten, a protein found in wheat, barley, rye, and triticale, severely damages the lining of the small intestine, leading to nutrient deficiencies, infertility, reduced bone density, and even some cancers. It may or may not be accompanied by neurological symptoms, weight loss, and digestive pain. The disease occurs in at least 1 percent of the population, 83 percent of whom remain undiagnosed. If you observe any of these symptoms or have a family member with celiac disease, it is important to get tested for celiac *before* eliminating gluten from your diet.

SATURATED AND OMEGA-6 FATS

Excess dietary intake of saturated fat and omega-6 fats has been linked to gut dysbiosis, whereas omega-3 fats and monounsaturated fats have a protective effect on the microbiota. However, many of the studies incriminating saturated fat to changes in the microbiota were performed on mice and used a feed containing half of total calories from sugar. Whether this effect would have been observed without the presence of sugar, using a whole foods paleo or "ancestral" diet, for example, is worth considering.

THICKENERS

Food emulsifiers, such as xanthan gum, guar gum, carrageenan, cellulose gum, and lecithin, have been linked to altered gut microbiota, bacterial overgrowth, intestinal permeability, inflammatory bowel disease, overweight, and metabolic syndrome. They are found in nearly all processed foods, including those that you probably think of as healthy, such as commercially prepared yogurts, low-fat products, almond milk, coconut milk, and gluten-free baked goods.

ALCOHOL

Excessive alcohol consumption is linked to changes in the gut microbiota, inflammation, impairment of gut and liver function, and increased risk for liver disease. However, moderate consumption of alcohol could have gut-protective effects. Research published in the *Natural Medicine Journal* in 2012 found that consuming up to two glasses of red wine daily over a period of 10 days decreased pathogenic bacteria among study participants and showed a prebiotic effect in concentrations of beneficial gut bacteria. Nevertheless, the vast majority of research implicates excessive alcohol consumption in an altered microbiome, not to mention numerous other health consequences. So, if you do choose to drink, choose fermented beverages such as wine, beer, and cider, and avoid liquor and sugary mixers.

SMOKING

It should go without saying that smoking tobacco products is detrimental to your health in myriad ways. Not surprisingly, it is also harmful to your microbiota. Fortunately, an overwhelming body of research indicates that quitting smoking causes profound and positive changes on the gut biome, increasing good bacteria and bacterial diversity.

ANTIBIOTICS

Antibiotic use significantly disrupts the gut microbiota, which is why many progressive health practitioners choose antibiotics as a last resort and advise patients to supplement antibiotic treatment with probiotics. A study published in the journal *PLoS One* in 2014 found that even a short course of antibiotics reduced bacterial diversity by 25 percent and reduced core phylogenetic microbiota by more than half. Because the drug does not distinguish between good bacteria and pathological bacteria, it has a devastating effect on the gut ecosystem.

NSAIDS

According to research published in the journal *Current Drug Safety*, nonsteroidal anti-inflammatory drugs (NSAIDs), such as aspirin, ibuprofen, and naproxen, "are responsible for a marked reduction of Lactobacilli, which act in the maintenance of luminal pH, mucosal permeability, enterocyte adhesion, mucus production, and immune system modulation." This adds to the mountains of evidence linking NSAIDs to intestinal damage.

CHEMICALS

Residual pesticides and herbicides found in conventionally grown foods may harm the microbiome, particularly glyphosate, the chemical in Roundup, the most commonly used herbicide in conventional farming. A 2013 article published in the journal *Entropy* argued that glyphosate inhibits enzymes and disrupts the biosynthesis of aromatic amino acids by gut bacteria, which may lead to gastrointestinal disorders, obesity, and numerous other chronic diseases.

Part Two

RECIPES FOR YOUR MICROBIOTA

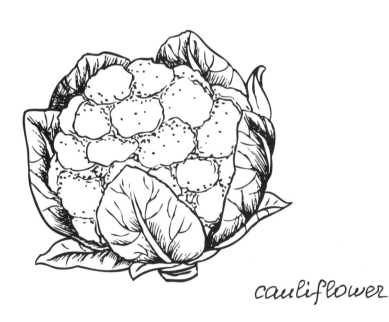

cauliflower

2

SALADS

Little Gem Lettuce with Goat Cheese and Figs

Mixed Greens in Moroccan Dressing

Tangled Vegetable Noodle Salad with Miso Vinaigrette

Mixed Greens with Pistachios and Grapefruit

Shaved Fennel, Microgreens, and Pomegranate

Radish, Arugula, and Feta Salad

Watermelon and Avocado Salad with Mint

Garlicky Kale Salad

Dandelion Greens with Balsamic Roasted Beets

Chilled Lentils, Cherries, and Basil

Potato Salad in White Wine Vinaigrette

Brussels Sprout and Apple Slaw with Apple Cider Vinaigrette

LITTLE GEM LETTUCE WITH GOAT CHEESE AND FIGS

Serves: 2 **Prep Time:** 5 minutes **Cook Time:** 0 minutes

Goat cheese is a tangy and delicious source of probiotics, and many people find it easier to digest than cow's milk dairy products. It pairs beautifully with prebiotic-rich sweet figs and raw honey.

2 tablespoons white wine vinegar

1 teaspoon raw honey

2 tablespoons extra-virgin olive oil

Sea salt

Freshly ground black pepper

4 heads little gem lettuce, cut into chunks

8 fresh figs, halved

4 ounces goat cheese, crumbled

1 In a large bowl, whisk together the vinegar, honey, and olive oil. Season to taste with salt and pepper.

2 Add the lettuce and fig halves to the bowl and toss gently to coat.

3 Divide the salad between serving plates and garnish with the crumbled goat cheese.

MIXED GREENS
IN MOROCCAN DRESSING

Serves: 2 to 4   **Prep Time:** 5 minutes   **Cook Time:** 0 minutes

The flavors in this salad are bold and border on overpowering. But to me, they're perfect. I love serving it with Falafel (page 34) and Hummus (page 118) for a complete meal. Paprika and garlic are naturally antimicrobial foods, and the lettuce and onion offer a healthy dose of prebiotics.

1 teaspoon anchovy paste

2 teaspoons minced garlic

1 teaspoon cumin seeds, roughly ground

1 teaspoon smoked paprika

Pinch cayenne pepper

¼ cup minced fresh flat-leaf parsley

2 tablespoons red wine vinegar

¼ cup extra-virgin olive oil

Sea salt

Freshly ground black pepper

8 cups mixed lettuces, hand torn into bite-size pieces

1 cup grape tomatoes, halved

1 small red onion, halved and thinly sliced

1 In a large bowl, whisk together the anchovy paste, garlic, cumin, paprika, cayenne, parsley, and vinegar. Slowly drizzle in the olive oil, whisking constantly to emulsify. Season to taste with salt and pepper.

2 Add the lettuce, tomatoes, and red onion to the bowl and toss gently to coat. Serve immediately.

TANGLED VEGETABLE NOODLE SALAD WITH MISO VINAIGRETTE

Serves: 2 to 4   **Prep Time:** 10 minutes   **Cook Time:** 0 minutes

This is my all-time favorite raw-vegan entrée salad. It's loaded with nutrients, and because it contains both prebiotics and probiotics, it's considered "symbiotic." Choose whatever dark leafy greens you like best, such as kale, chard, or mixed spring lettuces.

1 beet, unpeeled, with greens

2 carrots, unpeeled

2 cups roughly chopped dark leafy greens

½ cup hand-torn fresh basil leaves (optional)

2 tablespoons white miso

Juice of 1 lime

1 teaspoon minced fresh ginger

2 tablespoons low-sodium, gluten-free soy sauce

2 tablespoons extra-virgin olive oil

2 tablespoons toasted sesame oil

2 tablespoons hemp seeds

2 tablespoons pepitas

1 Use a spiralizer to make long curly noodles from the beet and carrots. If you do not have this tool, use a vegetable peeler to create long noodles from the carrot and julienne the beet with a sharp chef's knife.

2 Dice the beet stems finely and roughly chop the greens.

3 Toss the vegetable noodles with all of the greens, beet stems, and basil, if using. Set aside.

4 In a glass jar or measuring cup, whisk together the miso, lime juice, ginger, and soy sauce. Slowly drizzle in the oils, whisking constantly to form an emulsion. Pour the dressing over the salad and toss gently to coat.

5 Divide the salad between plates and shower with the hemp seeds and pepitas. Serve immediately.

MIXED GREENS WITH PISTACHIOS AND GRAPEFRUIT

Serves: 2   **Prep Time:** 10 minutes   **Cook Time:** 0 minutes

Pistachios are a lesser-known source of resistant starch and a good source of prebiotics. They add a delicious crunch and pretty color to this simple starter salad.

4 cups mixed baby greens

1 grapefruit

1 tablespoon white wine vinegar

1 teaspoon raw honey

Pinch sea salt

Freshly ground black pepper

2 tablespoons extra-virgin olive oil

¼ cup shelled, roughly chopped pistachios

1 Arrange the lettuce on serving plates.

2 Cut the ends off of the grapefruit using a paring knife, stand it on one end, and then cut away the peel. Carefully slice between the membranes to remove the grapefruit segments. Scatter the segments on and around the lettuce leaves.

3 In a small glass jar or measuring cup, whisk together the vinegar, honey, salt, and pepper. Slowly drizzle in the olive oil, whisking constantly to emulsify. Pour the dressing over the lettuce. Top with pistachios. Serve immediately.

SHAVED FENNEL, MICROGREENS, AND POMEGRANATE

Serves: 2 to 4   **Prep Time:** 10 minutes   **Cook Time:** 0 minutes

I never really think about the health benefits when I'm eating this salad—it just tastes so good! That said, each ingredient is a superfood in its own right and makes this side salad a nutritional powerhouse of antioxidants, polyphenols, and prebiotics. Top it with grilled chicken or crumbled tempeh to make it a main course.

½ fennel bulb, cored

2 cups microgreens

1 pomegranate, arils (seeds) removed

2 tablespoons balsamic vinegar

1 teaspoon raw honey

¼ cup extra-virgin olive oil

Sea salt

Freshly ground black pepper

1 Using a sharp chef's knife, cut the fennel bulb into paper-thin slices. Add them to a salad bowl along with the microgreens and pomegranate arils.

2 In a small glass jar or measuring cup, whisk together the vinegar and honey. Slowly drizzle in the olive oil, whisking constantly to emulsify. Season to taste with salt and pepper. Drizzle over the salad and toss very gently to coat. Serve immediately.

RADISH, ARUGULA, AND FETA SALAD

Serves: 4   **Prep Time:** 10 minutes   **Cook Time:** 0 minutes

Watermelon radishes are especially pretty in this peppery salad.

1 bunch radishes, thinly sliced

2 cups arugula

2 oranges, peeled and segmented

2 tablespoons white wine vinegar

1 teaspoon raw honey

¼ cup extra-virgin olive oil

Sea salt

Freshly ground black pepper

½ cup crumbled feta cheese

1 Combine the radishes, arugula, and orange segments in a large mixing bowl.

2 In a small glass jar, whisk together the vinegar, honey, and olive oil and season with salt and pepper. Pour the dressing over the salad and use your hands to gently toss. Spread the salad on a serving platter and top with the crumbled feta.

WATERMELON AND AVOCADO SALAD WITH MINT

Serves: 4   **Prep Time:** 5 minutes   **Cook Time:** 0 minutes

Watermelon and avocado are excellent sources of fermentable carbohydrates, which makes this delicious salad equally appealing for your microbiome. Prepare the salad just before you intend to serve it. For convenience, prepare the ingredients ahead and store them separately, and combine at the last minute.

6 cups cubed watermelon

2 avocados, diced

2 shallots, thinly sliced in rings

¼ cup roughly chopped mint leaves

Juice of 1 lime

Sea salt

Freshly ground black pepper

Combine the watermelon, avocado, shallots, mint, and lime juice in a large serving bowl. Season with salt and pepper. Serve immediately.

GARLICKY KALE SALAD

Serves: 2 to 4   **Prep Time:** 5 minutes   **Cook Time:** 0 minutes

This isn't exactly the salad you want to have moments before a big job interview. But all that garlic, not to mention the kale, is loaded with prebiotics. I like to use a Microplane grater to process the garlic because it produces a purée that disperses evenly throughout the dressing, coating each kale leaf.

4 to 6 garlic cloves, minced	Pinch sea salt
Zest and juice of 1 lemon	¼ cup extra-virgin olive oil
1 tablespoon red wine vinegar	1 bunch Lacinato kale
Pinch red chile flakes	1 small zucchini, julienned

1 In a large bowl, whisk together the garlic, lemon zest and juice, vinegar, chile flakes, and sea salt. Slowly drizzle in the olive oil, whisking constantly to emulsify.

2 Add the kale and use your hands to coat it thoroughly with the dressing. Add the zucchini and toss gently to mix. Divide between salad plates and serve immediately.

DANDELION GREENS WITH BALSAMIC ROASTED BEETS

Serves: 2 to 4   **Prep Time:** 10 minutes   **Cook Time:** 30 minutes

Roasted beets have a sweet, earthy flavor that offsets the slight bitterness of dandelion greens. Both are packed with prebiotics, not to mention a host of other micronutrients. If you want to serve this as a light entrée, add 2 ounces of goat cheese to each serving.

1 bunch beets, peeled, stems and greens reserved for another use

4 tablespoons extra-virgin olive oil, divided

3 tablespoons balsamic vinegar, divided

1 tablespoon raw honey

4 to 6 cups fresh dandelion greens, rinsed and patted dry

Sea salt

Freshly ground black pepper

1 Preheat the oven to 375°F. Cut the beets into quarters and spread out in a baking dish. Drizzle with 2 tablespoons of the olive oil and season with salt and pepper. Roast uncovered for 25 minutes. Add 2 tablespoons of the balsamic vinegar and the honey, tossing gently to coat. Roast for another 5 minutes.

2 In a large salad bowl, whisk together the remaining 2 tablespoons of olive oil and 1 tablespoon of balsamic vinegar. Season to taste with salt and pepper. Just before serving, add the dandelion greens and gently toss to coat in the dressing. Divide the greens between serving plates.

3 Divide the roasted beets between the salads. Spoon pan juices over each salad and serve immediately.

CHILLED LENTILS, CHERRIES, AND BASIL

Serves: 2 to 4   **Prep Time:** 10 minutes   **Cook Time:** 20 minutes

This tangy salad is delicious as an entrée or side salad. Make sure to add the cherries and basil just before serving. It will keep well in the refrigerator only if stored separately. If you want to make this salad in the wintertime when cherries aren't in season, use unsweetened dried cherries.

1 cup green lentils, rinsed and sorted

3 cups water

2 tablespoons red wine vinegar

2 tablespoons extra-virgin olive oil

2 cups halved, pitted fresh cherries

2 scallions, thinly sliced on a bias

1 cup hand-torn fresh basil leaves

Sea salt

Freshly ground black pepper

1 Place the lentils in a medium sauce pan with the water. Bring to a simmer over medium–low heat, cover, and cook until the lentils are tender but still slightly chewy, about 20 minutes. Drain in a colander and allow to cool briefly before placing in a serving dish.

2 Whisk together the vinegar and oil. Pour over the lentils and toss to combine. Add the cherries, scallions, and basil. Season with salt and pepper. Toss to combine and serve at room temperature.

POTATO SALAD IN WHITE WINE VINAIGRETTE

Serves: 4   **Prep Time:** 10 minutes   **Cook Time:** 25 minutes

Cooked and cooled potatoes are an excellent source of resistant starch, which feeds your healthy gut bacteria. When selecting pickles, make sure to purchase pickles with live, active cultures. They're available in the fresh, refrigerated section of the supermarket. Shelf-stable pasteurized pickles do not contain live bacterial cultures.

2 pounds Yukon gold or new potatoes, about 1½ inches in diameter

½ cup diced pickles

¼ cup minced fresh chives

3 tablespoons white wine vinegar

½ teaspoon Dijon mustard

Sea salt

Freshly ground black pepper

¼ cup extra-virgin olive oil

1 Place the potatoes in a large pot and cover with cold water. Bring to a boil over medium heat, cover, and cook for 25 minutes, until fork tender. Drain and allow to rest until cool enough to handle. Remove the peels from the potato, cut into 1-inch cubes, and place in a serving dish.

2 Add the pickles and chives to the potatoes.

3 In a small glass jar or measuring cup, whisk together the vinegar and mustard with salt and pepper. Slowly drizzle in the oil, whisking constantly to emulsify. Pour the dressing over the potatoes and toss very gently to coat. Serve at room temperature or allow to chill thoroughly before serving.

BRUSSELS SPROUT AND APPLE SLAW WITH APPLE CIDER VINAIGRETTE

Serves: 4   **Prep Time:** 10 minutes   **Cook Time:** 0 minutes

Brussels sprouts and apples are rich sources of prebiotics, so much so that a little goes a long way, and too much may cause digestive discomfort. Enjoy as a side salad or add a few ounces of grilled chicken or fish to make a complete meal.

1 pound brussels sprouts

1 Granny Smith or Braeburn apple

3 tablespoons apple cider vinegar

1 teaspoon raw honey

¼ cup extra-virgin olive oil

Sea salt

Freshly ground black pepper

½ cup unsweetened dried cherries (optional)

1 Cut the tough, woody ends from the bottom of each brussels sprout and peel away any discolored outer leaves. Run the sprouts through the slicing attachment of a food processor (not the shredder or the usual blade) to produce a slaw. Core the apple and process it in the same manner.

2 In a large bowl, whisk together the vinegar and honey. Slowly drizzle in the olive oil, whisking constantly to emulsify. Season to taste with salt and pepper.

3 Add the shredded brussels sprouts and apple to the bowl and toss to mix thoroughly. Stir in the dried cherries, if using, and serve immediately.

3

APPETIZERS & SIDES

Goat Cheese and Cauliflower Fritters

Salad Rolls

Falafel

Greek Broccoli Couscous

Grilled Vegetable Platter with Citrus and Garlic

Smokey Stewed Kale

Red Cabbage and Apples

Creamed Broccoli

Sweet Potato Gratin with Rosemary and Pecans

Wild Rice and Cranberry Pilaf

Caribbean Rice and Bean Salad

Quinoa and Avocado Salad

GOAT CHEESE
AND CAULIFLOWER FRITTERS

Serves: 2 to 4   **Prep Time:** 10 minutes   **Cook Time:** 20 minutes

These tangy little fritters offer the perfect balance of sweet, sour, and savory. They also make a delicious entrée when served with a simple side salad. Cauliflower and pomegranate are rich sources of prebiotics, and goat cheese and yogurt offer probiotics. If you prefer an alternative to coconut flour, use ½ cup of a gluten-free flour blend, or wheat flour if it is tolerable.

1 head cauliflower, broken into florets

4 ounces crumbled goat cheese

¼ cup roughly chopped fresh flat-leaf parsley

2 shallots, minced

Zest of 1 lemon

1 egg, whisked

¼ cup coconut flour

1 teaspoon baking powder

Sea salt

2 tablespoons coconut oil

½ cup Plain Yogurt (page 68)

1 tablespoon lemon juice

1 teaspoon ground sumac, plus more for serving

1½ cups Pomegranate Gremolata (page 117)

1 Bring a large pot of salted water to a boil. Also prepare an ice-water bath in a large bowl. Blanch the cauliflower in the boiling water until nearly tender, about 5 minutes. Plunge into the ice-water bath, drain, and add to a large food processor. Pulse until crumbly.

2 Add the goat cheese, parsley, shallots, lemon zest, egg, flour, baking powder, and a generous pinch of salt to the food processor. Pulse until just combined.

3 Melt the coconut oil in a large skillet over medium heat. Form the cauliflower mixture into small patties. Fry on each side for 2 to 3 minutes, or until a brown crust develops. Flip and cook on the other side. Set aside in a warmed oven while you finish with the remainder of the mixture.

4 While the fritters are cooking, whisk the yogurt, lemon juice, and sumac together. Set aside.

5 Set two fritters on a serving plate and top with the Pomegranate Gremolata, drizzle with yogurt mixture, and finish with a pinch of sumac.

SALAD ROLLS

Serves: 2   **Prep Time:** 15 minutes   **Cook Time:** 0 minutes

Most salad rolls are filled with rice noodles, but this version uses bean sprouts instead. Make sure to look for fresh sprouts without any "off" appearance or smell.

16 rice paper wrappers

2 cups mung bean sprouts

½ cup roughly chopped fresh cilantro

1 cucumber, peeled and cut into 4-inch long spears

2 carrots, peeled and grated

1 cup Peanut Sauce (page 121) or Sweet Chili Garlic Sauce (page 122), for serving.

1 Before beginning, assemble all of the ingredients so that you're ready to work quickly after soaking each rice paper wrapper.

2 Bring a pot of salted water to a simmer. Pour the water into a round pan large enough to accommodate the rice paper wrappers.

3 Place one of the wrappers into the water for about 10 seconds to soften. Remove it to a dry work surface and layer bean sprouts, cilantro, cucumber, and carrots in the center. Fold one side of the wrapper over the ingredients, tucking it under them. Fold in each end, and then roll to seal it shut.

4 Fill all of the salad rolls and serve immediately or refrigerate for up to 4 hours before serving. Serve with Peanut Sauce or Sweet Chili Garlic Sauce.

FALAFEL

Serves: 2 to 4   **Prep Time:** 10 minutes, plus 8 hours inactive time
Cook Time: 10 minutes

The first time I tried this recipe was when my second son was born and my friend Elizabeth brought us a meal. I couldn't believe it didn't contain any wheat and instantly fell in love with the vegan recipe, which she graciously shared with me. It can be served as an appetizer or with pita, tabbouleh, and a side salad for a complete meal.

1½ cups dried chickpeas

1 cup diced onion

2 garlic cloves, minced

½ cup minced fresh cilantro

1 tablespoon minced fresh mint

1 tablespoon lemon juice

1 teaspoon ground cumin

½ teaspoon sea salt

¼ teaspoon freshly ground black pepper

¼ cup coconut oil

1 cup Hummus (page 118), for serving

1 cup halved grape tomatoes, for serving

1 Soak the chickpeas in several cups of fresh water for 8 hours or overnight.

2 Thoroughly rinse and drain them and place in a food processor along with the onion, garlic, cilantro, mint, lemon juice, cumin, salt, and pepper. Pulse until nearly smooth, about the texture of cookie dough.

3 Heat the coconut oil in a large skillet over medium heat until hot. Form the chickpea mixture into small balls or patties and fry on all sides until golden brown. Set on a cooking rack set over a sheet pan to allow excess oil to drain. You can keep this in a warmed oven to keep the falafel hot while you finish with the remainder of the mixture.

4 Serve with hummus and grape tomatoes.

GREEK BROCCOLI COUSCOUS

Serves: 2   **Prep Time:** 5 minutes   **Cook Time:** 0 minutes

Couscous is made with wheat, which is high in carbs, and many people find it harmful to their gut. This version is made with broccoli, and the texture is remarkably similar.

1 head broccoli

Sea salt

Freshly ground black pepper

1 tablespoon olive oil

8 pitted kalamata olives

1 tablespoon minced fresh oregano

2 garlic cloves, minced

2 plum tomatoes, diced

¼ cup minced fresh flat-leaf parsley

Zest and juice of 1 lemon

1 Break the broccoli into large florets and put them into a food processor fitted with the standard blade. Pulse until it is coarsely chopped and resembles couscous.

2 Place the broccoli into a large bowl and season with salt and pepper. Add the olive oil, olives, oregano, garlic, tomatoes, parsley, and lemon zest and juice. Toss to mix. Allow the salad to rest for at least 10 minutes to allow the flavors to come together. Serve chilled.

GRILLED VEGETABLE PLATTER WITH CITRUS AND GARLIC

Serves: 4   **Prep Time:** 5 minutes   **Cook Time:** 1 hour

This festive platter is so full of flavor. You can certainly substitute whatever vegetable is available and in season at the time. The cook time is lengthy, but you can save time by roasting the garlic a day ahead. Leftovers make great additions to your morning omelet.

1 head garlic

¼ cup olive oil, divided

¼ teaspoon sea salt

2 tablespoons lime juice

2 tablespoons orange juice

1 red bell pepper, cored and halved

1 medium eggplant, cut into eighths lengthwise

2 small zucchini, cut into quarters lengthwise

1 Preheat the oven to 350°F. Slice the top off the head of garlic and place it on a square of foil. Drizzle with 1 teaspoon of olive oil. Fold the foil over the garlic and wrap loosely into a small package. Roast for 35 to 45 minutes. This step can be done up to a day ahead of time. When the garlic is cool enough to handle, squeeze each of the cloves out of the papery garlic skins.

2 Mash the roasted garlic together with the salt, lime juice, orange juice, and all but 1 teaspoon of the remaining olive oil in a mortar and pestle or blend in a blender until a smooth paste is formed.

3 Heat an outdoor gas or charcoal grill or heat a grill pan to medium heat.

4 Coat the skin side of the pepper halves with the remaining teaspoon of olive oil. Roast the red pepper skin side down over the highest heat section of the grill. When charred, remove to a covered container to steam. Peel off the skin then slice the roasted peppers into thin strips.

5 Spread the garlic paste on the cut sides of the eggplant and zucchini. Place the eggplant and zucchini skin side down and cook for 2 to 3 minutes, until blistered but not charred. Turn the vegetables to cook on the other side for 2 minutes; turn again and cook for another 2 minutes.

6 Serve the vegetables on a platter family style.

SMOKY STEWED KALE

Serves: 2 to 4   **Prep Time:** 5 minutes   **Cook Time:** 35 minutes

Kale and garlic are rich in prebiotics, and the apple cider vinegar offers a nice dose of probiotics. I prefer to enjoy kale either raw and crunchy, or stewed over moderate heat until it's meltingly tender. This side dish is decidedly in the latter category. I usually enjoy it with a simple roasted chicken.

2 tablespoons olive oil

2 garlic cloves, minced

1 yellow onion, minced

1 tablespoon smoked paprika

2 tablespoons tomato paste

1 cup diced tomatoes, either fresh or canned

8 cups Lacinato kale, stems minced, leaves roughly chopped

1 cup vegetable broth or Chicken Bone Broth (page 57)

1 tablespoon apple cider vinegar

Sea salt

Freshly ground black pepper

1 Heat the oil in a large skillet over medium heat. Add the garlic and onion and cook for about 5 to 7 minutes, until soft and translucent.

2 Add the paprika, tomato paste, and diced tomatoes. Cook for 3 minutes.

3 Add the kale and broth and simmer uncovered for 25 minutes, stirring occasionally.

4 Remove from the heat and stir in the apple cider vinegar. Season with salt and pepper.

RED CABBAGE AND APPLES

Serves: 2 to 4   **Prep Time:** 5 minutes   **Cook Time:** 5 to 7 minutes

This side dish is the perfect accompaniment to roasted pork chops or pan-seared fish.

1 head red cabbage, cored and shredded

2 apples, cored and thinly sliced into wedges

1 teaspoon ground cloves (optional)

1 tablespoon extra-virgin olive oil

Sea salt

Freshly ground black pepper

1 tablespoon apple cider vinegar

1 Combine the cabbage, apples, cloves, and olive oil in a large sauce pan. Season with salt and pepper. Cover and cook on low for 5 to 7 minutes, or until the cabbage is bright and tender.

2 Add the apple cider vinegar and toss to combine. Serve immediately.

CREAMED BROCCOLI

Serves: 2   **Prep Time:** 5 minutes   **Cook Time:** 20 minutes

I find mushy vegetables surprisingly comforting. Simmering vegetables gently over low heat allows their complex and sometimes overpowering flavors to become soft and sweet. Make sure to remove the broccoli from the heat before you stir in the yogurt. This ensures it doesn't curdle or damage the healthy bacteria.

1 tablespoon extra-virgin olive oil

3 garlic cloves, minced

Pinch red chile flakes

1 head broccoli, cut into florets

1 cup vegetable broth or Chicken Bone Broth (page 57)

½ cup full-fat Greek yogurt, at room temperature

Sea salt

Freshly ground black pepper

1 Heat the olive oil in a large skillet over medium–low heat. Add the garlic, chile flakes, and broccoli. Cook for about 2 minutes.

2 Pour in the broth, cover, and cook for 20 minutes.

3 Remove the broccoli from the heat. Use an immersion blender to purée until somewhat smooth. Stir in the yogurt and season with salt and pepper.

SWEET POTATO GRATIN WITH ROSEMARY AND PECANS

Serves: 4 to 6   **Prep Time:** 10 minutes
Cook Time: 1 hour 20 minutes

I made this delicious gratin for Thanksgiving one year as a healthy alternative to the traditional marshmallow-topped side dish. It was even better than the original and so much better for us. I also loved being able to prepare the entire dish ahead of time and set it in the refrigerator to rest until I was ready to cook it. Leave the sweet potatoes unpeeled when you boil them for minimal nutrient loss.

4 large sweet potatoes

Sea salt

¼ cup butter, ghee, or coconut oil, melted

½ cup roughly chopped pecans

1 tablespoon minced fresh rosemary

1 Place the sweet potatoes in a large pot, cover with water, and add a generous pinch of sea salt. Cover and bring to a boil over medium heat. Simmer for 20 minutes. Drain the sweet potatoes and allow to rest until cool enough to handle.

2 Preheat the oven to 350°F.

3 Remove the peels and slice the sweet potatoes into ¼-inch rounds.

4 Coat the interior of a 4-quart baking dish with 1 teaspoon of the butter. Place the sweet potato rounds into the dish. Top with a drizzle of butter, a sprinkle of pecans, and a pinch of rosemary.

5 Repeat with the remaining sweet potatoes, butter, pecans, and rosemary. Cover the dish with aluminum foil.

6 Bake for 45 minutes. Remove the foil and continue baking for another 10 to 15 minutes, until all of the sweet potatoes are fork tender and beginning to brown around the edges.

WILD RICE
AND CRANBERRY PILAF

Serves: 4   **Prep Time:** 5 minutes   **Cook Time:** 45 to 55 minutes

Wild rice is a good source of fiber and is rich in magnesium, which improves muscle contraction and relaxation, allowing for healthy digestion. Look for fruit-juice sweetened or unsweetened dried cranberries to avoid added sugars.

1 cup wild rice

4 cups vegetable broth or Chicken Bone Broth (page 57)

½ cup dried cranberries

2 green onions (green parts only) thinly sliced

1 teaspoon minced fresh sage

1 tablespoon balsamic vinegar

Sea salt

Freshly ground black pepper

1 In a medium pot, bring the wild rice and broth to a simmer over medium heat. Cover, turn the heat to low, and simmer for 45 to 55 minutes, until all of the liquid is absorbed. Fluff with a fork.

2 Stir in the cranberries, green onions, sage, and balsamic vinegar. Season with salt and pepper.

3 Serve warm or chilled.

CARIBBEAN RICE AND BEAN SALAD

Serves: 4   **Prep Time:** 10 minutes   **Cook Time:** 20 minutes

This recipe is adapted from the *Moosewood Restaurant Celebrates* cookbook, one of my favorite vegetarian cookbooks. White rice is a good source of resistant starch and is more easily digestible than brown rice. However, if you prefer the added fiber, use brown rice and double the water and cooking time.

1 cup white rice

1½ cups water

¼ cup lime juice

2 tablespoons extra-virgin olive oil

¼ cup minced flat-leaf parsley

¼ cup minced fresh cilantro

1 teaspoon fresh thyme

1 teaspoon smoked paprika

2 green onions (white and green parts) thinly sliced on a bias

1 red bell pepper, cored, seeded, and diced

1 cup cooked black beans, rinsed and drained

Sea salt

Freshly ground black pepper

1 Bring the rice to a simmer in a small pot along with the water and a pinch of sea salt. Cover and cook on low heat until tender, about 20 minutes. Fluff with a fork.

2 In a glass jar or measuring cup, whisk together the lime juice, olive oil, parsley, cilantro, thyme, and paprika. Season to taste with salt and pepper.

3 Add the green onions, bell pepper, and black beans to the rice. Pour the dressing over the top and toss gently to combine. Serve at room temperature or chill thoroughly before serving.

QUINOA AND AVOCADO SALAD

Serves: 4   **Prep Time:** 10 minutes   **Cook Time:** 20 minutes

This salad is loaded with prebiotics and filling protein and fiber, making it an awesome vegan entrée or a great side dish to take to summer potlucks or barbecues.

1 cup quinoa, rinsed and drained

1¼ cups vegetable broth or Chicken Bone Broth (page 57)

2 garlic cloves, minced

Zest and juice of 2 limes

2 tablespoons olive oil

Sea salt

Freshly ground black pepper

1 cup roughly chopped fresh cilantro

1 pint grape tomatoes, halved

2 avocados, cored and diced

2 green onions (white and green parts) thinly sliced on a bias

1 (15-ounce) can black beans, rinsed and drained

1 In a medium pot, bring the quinoa to a simmer over low heat with the broth. Cover and cook until tender, about 20 minutes. Fluff with a fork.

2 In a glass jar or measuring cup, combine the garlic, lime zest and juice, and olive oil. Season to taste with salt and pepper.

3 Add the cilantro, tomatoes, avocado, green onions, and black beans to the quinoa. Pour the dressing over the entire mixture and toss very gently to combine. Serve at room temperature or chill thoroughly. If you plan to wait more than 1 hour until serving, add the avocado just prior to serving.

4

SOUPS & BONE BROTHS

Raw Avocado Bisque

Watermelon Gazpacho

Chilled Borscht

Chard and Potato Stew

Vichyssoise

Butternut Squash Bisque

Roasted Garlic and Creamy Cauliflower Bisque

Kale and White Bean Stew

Beef and Rice Soup

Indonesian Laksa

Chicken Bone Broth

Beef Bone Broth

RAW AVOCADO BISQUE

Serves: 2 to 4   **Prep Time:** 10 minutes   **Cook Time:** 0 minutes

Avocados are a good source of polyols, fermentable carbohydrates that are part of a larger group of carbohydrates known as FODMAPs. Avocado also contains nourishing monounsaturated fats. Add some shallots, garlic, tomatoes, cucumber, and cilantro, and this soup is like an energy drink for your microbiota.

2 ripe avocados, peeled and pitted

1 cucumber, peeled and diced

1 shallot, minced

1 small garlic clove, minced

1 cup roughly chopped fresh cilantro, divided

¼ cup extra-virgin olive oil

1 tablespoon apple cider vinegar

Sea salt

Freshly ground pepper

½ cup seeded, diced tomato

1 Place the avocado, cucumber, shallot, garlic, and all but 2 tablespoons of the cilantro in a blender. Pour in the olive oil and apple cider vinegar.

2 Purée until completely smooth. Season to taste with salt and pepper.

3 To serve, garnish each portion of soup with diced tomato and the remaining cilantro.

WATERMELON GAZPACHO

Serves: 2 to 4   **Prep Time:** 10 minutes   **Cook Time:** 0 minutes

Watermelon is another good source of fermentable carbohydrates, specifically fructose. The soup is best in summertime when watermelon is ripe and sweet, its flavors beautifully offset by the mild heat of Fresno chile.

2 cups cubed seedless watermelon

4 cups seeded, diced tomatoes, divided

1 cucumber, peeled and diced, divided

½ Fresno chile, seeded and minced

2 tablespoons extra-virgin olive oil

2 tablespoons red wine vinegar

¼ cup roughly chopped fresh cilantro

1 shallot, minced

Sea salt

Freshly ground black pepper

1   Place the watermelon, 2 cups of tomatoes, half of the cucumber, chile, olive oil, and vinegar into a blender and pulse until mostly smooth.

2   Stir in the remaining tomatoes and cucumber along with the cilantro and shallot. Season to taste with salt and pepper.

CHILLED BORSCHT

Serves: 2 to 4   **Prep Time:** 10 minutes   **Cook Time:** 20 minutes

Beets and cabbage are excellent sources of prebiotics, especially when they're gently cooked. This soup can be enjoyed hot or cold. If you prefer a vegan soup, use the vegetable broth.

1 bunch beets, peeled and diced

1 shallot, minced

1 garlic clove, minced

1 cup shredded red cabbage

1 carrot, peeled and shredded

1 celery stalk, minced

1 thyme sprig

⅛ teaspoon ground allspice

2 cups vegetable broth or Chicken Bone Broth (page 57)

Sea salt

Freshly ground black pepper

1 bunch fresh dill, roughly chopped, for serving

1 lemon, cut into wedges, for serving

1 Combine the beets, shallot, garlic, cabbage, carrot, celery, thyme, allspice, and broth in a large pot and bring to a simmer. Cover and cook on low for 20 minutes. Season to taste with salt and pepper. Remove the thyme sprig.

2 Remove the soup from the heat and chill thoroughly, uncovered.

3 Garnish with fresh dill and lemon wedges.

CHARD AND POTATO STEW

Serves: 2 to 4   **Prep Time:** 10 minutes
Cook Time: 35 to 45 minutes

This hearty stew is loaded with prebiotics drenched in gut-nourishing bone broth.

2 tablespoons extra-virgin olive oil

1 yellow onion, diced

2 garlic cloves, smashed

1 (15-ounce) can plum tomatoes

2 thyme sprigs

Pinch red chile flakes

1 quart (4 cups) Chicken Bone Broth (page 57)

1 pound potatoes, peeled and diced

1 bunch Swiss chard, stems diced and leaves roughly chopped

Sea salt

Freshly ground black pepper

1 Heat the oil in a large pot over medium heat. Cook the onion and garlic until soft, about 10 minutes. Add the tomatoes, thyme, and red chile flakes. Cook for another 5 minutes.

2 Pour in the broth, and add the potatoes and chard. Simmer uncovered for 25 to 30 minutes, until the potatoes and chard are very soft. Season to taste with salt and pepper.

VICHYSSOISE

Serves: 4 **Prep Time:** 10 minutes **Cook Time:** 45 to 50 minutes

Leeks, onion, garlic, and potatoes marry beautifully in this creamy, comforting soup. It can be served hot, or chill it for a generous dose of resistant starch from the potatoes. Traditionally the soup is made with heavy cream, but you can also use coconut cream if you find dairy difficult to digest.

2 tablespoons extra-virgin olive oil

2 leeks, white and pale green parts only, halved and thinly sliced

1 yellow onion, diced

4 garlic cloves, smashed

1 pound yellow potatoes, peeled and diced

2 thyme sprigs

1 quart (4 cups) low-sodium vegetable broth or Chicken Bone Broth (page 57)

¼ cup heavy cream or coconut cream

Sea salt

Freshly ground black pepper

1 Heat the oil in a large pot over medium heat. Cook the leeks, onion, and garlic until soft, about 15 minutes. Add the potatoes and cook for another 5 minutes.

2 Add the thyme and pour in the broth. Cover and simmer for 25 to 30 minutes, until the potatoes are very soft. Add the heavy cream and stir until integrated.

3 Remove 2 cups of the soup to a blender and purée until completely smooth. Return the purée to the soup. Season to taste with salt and pepper.

BUTTERNUT SQUASH BISQUE

Serves: 4 to 6   **Prep Time:** 10 minutes   **Cook Time:** 40 minutes

This creamy, spicy butternut squash soup is delicious and warming in the winter. Serve with a dollop of Greek yogurt for an added bonus of probiotics.

1 tablespoon extra-virgin olive oil

1 yellow onion, diced

1 tablespoon minced ginger

1 tablespoon minced garlic

1 medium butternut squash, peeled, seeded, and cubed

1 quart (4 cups) Chicken Bone Broth (page 57)

1 tablespoon yellow curry powder

Sea salt

Freshly ground black pepper

½ cup full-fat Greek Yogurt (page 70), for serving

1 Heat the oil in a large pot over medium heat. Cook the onion, ginger, and garlic until soft, about 10 minutes.

2 Add the butternut squash, broth, and curry powder and bring to a simmer. Season with salt and pepper. Cook uncovered for about 30 minutes, until the squash is very tender. Purée with an immersion blender. Adjust the seasoning to taste with salt and pepper.

3 Serve with a generous spoonful of Greek yogurt.

ROASTED GARLIC AND CREAMY CAULIFLOWER BISQUE

Serves: 4   **Prep Time:** 10 minutes   **Cook Time:** 1 to 1¼ hours

Roasted garlic is so simple to make but adds complexity and richness to any dish, especially this creamy soup. If you can tolerate wheat, you can also use sourdough bread crumbs in place of the gluten-free bread crumbs.

1 head garlic

2 tablespoons extra-virgin olive oil, divided

1 head cauliflower, broken into florets

1 quart (4 cups) Chicken Bone Broth (page 57)

2 fresh thyme sprigs

Sea salt

Freshly ground black pepper

¼ cup minced fresh flat-leaf parsley

1 cup gluten-free bread crumbs

1 Preheat the oven to 350°F. Slice the top off of the head of garlic and discard. Place the garlic on a square of foil. Drizzle with 1 tablespoon of the olive oil and wrap the foil into a loose package. Roast for 35 to 45 minutes, until the garlic is soft and fragrant. Remove the foil and allow the garlic to rest until it is cool enough to handle.

2 About halfway through cooking the garlic, place the cauliflower in a large pot along with the broth and thyme. Season with salt and pepper. Bring to a simmer, cover, and cook for 20 minutes.

3 When the garlic is cool enough to handle, squeeze the cloves from their papery skins and mash into a paste, reserving 2 cloves for the bread crumbs. Add the garlic paste to the cauliflower. Continue cooking until the cauliflower is soft, about another 10 to 15 minutes.

4 Remove the thyme sprig. Purée the soup with an immersion blender until smooth.

5 While the soup is cooking, preheat the broiler. Mash the remaining two garlic cloves with the remaining 1 tablespoon of oil. Toss it with the parsley and bread crumbs and spread them on a sheet pan. Toast under the broiler for 1 to 2 minutes, or until lightly browned and bubbling.

6 Divide the puréed soup between serving bowls and garnish with the toasted bread crumbs.

KALE AND WHITE BEAN STEW

Serves: 4   **Prep Time:** 10 minutes   **Cook Time:** 25 to 30 minutes

Despite its fading popularity, kale is my favorite dark leafy green. It's brimming with prebiotics, vitamins, and minerals. Beans are a good source of prebiotics as well. To make them more easily digestible, purchase dry beans and soak overnight before cooking in fresh water until tender.

1 tablespoon extra-virgin olive oil

1 onion, diced

2 carrots, unpeeled, diced

2 celery stalks, diced

4 garlic cloves, minced

Sea salt

1 quart (4 cups) vegetable broth or Chicken Bone Broth (page 57)

1 teaspoon fresh thyme

½ teaspoon minced fresh rosemary

1 bunch kale, stems diced, leaves roughly chopped

1 (15-ounce) can cannellini beans, rinsed and drained

1 Heat the olive oil in a large pot over medium heat. Cook the onion, carrots, celery, and garlic with a generous pinch of sea salt until tender, 10 to 15 minutes.

2 Add the broth, thyme, rosemary, kale, and beans. Cover and cook on low until the kale is tender, about 15 minutes.

BEEF AND RICE SOUP

Serves: 4 to 6   **Prep Time:** 10 minutes   **Cook Time:** 2½ to 3 hours

This simple, hearty soup is loaded with flavor and nutrients from the delicious beef bone broth. I use coconut oil because it is more heat stable for browning the meat than is olive oil.

1 tablespoon coconut oil

1 pound beef stew meat, cut into 1-inch cubes

Sea salt

Freshly ground black pepper

1 yellow onion, diced

2 carrots, diced

2 celery stalks, diced

2 garlic cloves, smashed

¼ cup dry sherry or red wine

1 bay leaf

1 cup brown rice

1 quart (4 cups) Beef Bone Broth (page 58)

1 Heat the coconut oil in a large pot over medium–high heat. Pat the beef cubes dry. Season generously with salt and pepper. Sear them in batches for a minute or two on each side to brown the exterior. Remove the meat to a separate dish.

2 Reduce the heat to medium. In the same pot, cook the onion, carrots, celery, and garlic until soft, about 10 minutes. Deglaze the pan with sherry or wine. Add the bay leaf, rice, broth, and the browned beef stew meat along with any juices that have accumulated in the dish.

3 Bring to a simmer, cover, and cook over medium-low heat for 2 to 2½ hours, until the beef is tender.

INDONESIAN LAKSA

Serves: 4   **Prep Time:** 10 minutes   **Cook Time:** 25 minutes

Laksa is a Southeast Asian noodle soup in a coconut broth. The primary ingredients and spices vary regionally. If you can find fresh lemon basil at your local farmer's market, definitely pick some up. It has an exquisite aroma and flavor that brightens everything from raw watermelon to savory grilled burgers. A combination of fresh cilantro and basil is a fine substitution.

4 ounces thin rice vermicelli

1 tablespoon coconut oil

1 yellow onion, halved and thinly sliced

1 tablespoon minced ginger

1 tablespoon minced garlic

1 teaspoon minced lemongrass

1 red bell pepper, cored and thinly sliced

1 quart (4 cups) Chicken Bone Broth (page 57)

1 teaspoon ground turmeric

1 (15-ounce) can coconut milk

Sea salt

Freshly ground black pepper

2 boneless, skinless chicken breasts, very thinly sliced

½ cup loosely packed lemon basil leaves

1 lime, cut into wedges, for serving

Sambal or other chili paste, for serving

1   Cover the rice vermicelli with cold water. Set aside and allow to rehydrate.

2   Heat the oil in a large pot over medium heat. Cook the onion, ginger, garlic, and lemongrass until slightly softened and fragrant, about 5 minutes.

3   Add the bell pepper, chicken broth, turmeric, and coconut milk and bring to a simmer. Season with salt and pepper. Cook uncovered for about 10 minutes.

4   Stir in the sliced chicken and simmer until just cooked through, about 10 minutes. Drain the vermicelli and stir into the soup. Allow to cook until just heated through. Stir in the lemon basil.

5   Serve with fresh lime wedges and sambal.

CHICKEN BONE BROTH

Yields: 1 quart (4 cups)   **Prep Time:** 5 minutes
Cook Time: 2 to 3 hours

Bone broth contains nourishing micronutrients to help repair a leaky gut and support a healthy digestive system. Save chicken bones from a whole roasted chicken and make the broth immediately, or store the bones in the freezer until you're ready to make it. The vinegar helps draw nutrients from the bones, as does the cold water.

1 pound chicken bones

1 tablespoon apple cider vinegar

1 teaspoon sea salt

2 quarts (8 cups) cold water

Place the chicken bones in a large pot. Add the vinegar, salt, and water. Bring to a simmer and cook, partially covered, over low heat for 2 to 3 hours until fragrant and savory. Use immediately or allow to cool before straining and placing into a container for storage. Refrigerate for up to 5 days. Freeze for up to 3 months.

BEEF BONE BROTH

Yields: 1 quart (4 cups)   **Prep Time:** 5 minutes
Cook Time: 3½ to 4½ hours

Make sure to roast the beef bones ahead of time before making this broth. It improves the flavor significantly.

1 pound beef bones

1 tablespoon apple cider vinegar

1 teaspoon sea salt

2 quarts (8 cups) water

1 Preheat the oven to 375°F. Spread the beef bones out on a sheet pan. Roast uncovered for 30 minutes.

2 Place the bones in a large pot. Add the vinegar, salt, and water. Bring to a simmer and cook, partially covered, for 3 to 4 hours. Use immediately or allow to cool before straining and placing into a container for storage. Refrigerate for up to 5 days. Freeze for up to 3 months.

5

JUICES & SMOOTHIES

Green Juice

Ginger Beet Juice

Tomato Celery Juice

Celery Apple Juice

Pineapple Cilantro Juice

Watercress Pear Juice

Kale Lime Pie Smoothie

Banana Almond Butter Smoothie

Detoxifying Green Smoothie

Cherry Cheesecake Smoothie

Triple Berry Smoothie

Mint Chocolate Smoothie

GREEN JUICE

Serves: 2   **Prep Time:** 5 minutes   **Cook Time:** 0 minutes

My friend Shireen says that juice gives her everything she wanted from coffee. Once I started juicing, I understood what she meant. It gave me boundless energy! One of the reasons for this is the enzymes present in raw fruit and vegetables. This is the green juice recipe I come back to again and again.

6 celery stalks

2 apples, halved

2 lemons or limes, peeled

1 bunch kale

Run all of the ingredients through a juicer. Enjoy immediately.

GINGER BEET JUICE

Serves: 2   **Prep Time:** 5 minutes   **Cook Time:** 0 minutes

Beets have a strong, earthy flavor, but I find it almost completely masked by the ginger in this classic juice recipe. I like to use the beet greens and stems as well, but you can skip them if you prefer. They dull the brilliant red hue of the juice slightly, but improve its nutritional profile.

1 bunch beets

4 carrots

1 sweet apple, such as Fuji or Pink Lady, halved

2 lemons, peeled

2-inch knob ginger

Run all of the ingredients through a juicer. Enjoy immediately.

TOMATO CELERY JUICE

Serves: 2   **Prep Time:** 5 minutes   **Cook Time:** 0 minutes

This might just remind you of your favorite cocktail, but so much healthier and brilliantly fresh. Keep it healthy and skip the booze. If you choose a conventionally grown cucumber, peel it before running through your juicer.

4 celery stalks

8 ripe tomatoes

1 cucumber

1 small lemon, peeled

Pinch cayenne pepper

Pinch sea salt

Run the celery, tomatoes, cucumber, and lemon through a juicer. Stir in the cayenne and sea salt. Enjoy immediately.

CELERY APPLE JUICE

Serves: 2 to 4   **Prep Time:** 5 minutes   **Cook Time:** 0 minutes

I first enjoyed this juice at a farmer's market in Phoenix. Since then, I've loved the combination of apple and celery.

6 to 8 celery stalks

4 tart apples, such as Granny Smith, halved

½ bunch fresh flat-leaf parsley

1 lemon

Run all of the ingredients through a juicer. Enjoy immediately.

PINEAPPLE CILANTRO JUICE

Serves: 2 to 4   **Prep Time:** 5 minutes   **Cook Time:** 0 minutes

Someday I'll write a cookbook devoted to cilantro. I just love it—especially when combined with pineapple and citrus. This recipe calls for a whole pineapple, so you may wish to split this juice among four servings to avoid consuming all of that sugar.

1 pineapple, peeled and cut into spears

1 bunch fresh cilantro

1 lime, peeled

1 orange, peeled

Run all of the ingredients through a juicer. Enjoy immediately.

WATERCRESS PEAR JUICE

Serves: 2   **Prep Time:** 5 minutes   **Cook Time:** 0 minutes

This recipe is adapted from the cookbook *Living Raw Food* by Sarma Melngailis. While watercress might not normally find its way into your grocery basket, it should. It's brimming with antioxidants, vitamins, and minerals, which help heal oxidative stress and inflammation caused by processed foods. If you choose a conventionally grown cucumber, peel it before running through your juicer.

1 bunch watercress

1 cucumber

2 pears, unpeeled

2 limes, peeled

2 cups pineapple (about a quarter of a whole pineapple)

Run all of the ingredients through a juicer. Enjoy immediately.

KALE LIME PIE SMOOTHIE

Serves: 2   **Prep Time:** 5 minutes   **Cook Time:** 0 minutes

The first time I made this smoothie, I was undone. It tastes like a sweet tart made love to key lime pie. But with no sugar and a healthy dose of micronutrients, it's much better for you than either of those baked goods. If you do not have a juicer, simply place the ingredients in a blender and purée until smooth. Although I prefer the texture of the original version, the latter contains more prebiotics and fiber.

1 bunch fresh kale

2 limes, peeled

½ to 1 cup unsweetened almond milk

2 frozen bananas, cut into chunks

1 Run the kale and limes through a juicer. Place the juice into a high-speed blender along with the almond milk and banana chunks. Blend until smooth. Enjoy immediately.

IF YOU DO NOT HAVE A JUICER:

1 Remove the ribs from the kale and set aside for another use. Place the kale leaves, limes, and ½ cup of almond milk into a blender. Purée until very smooth, adding more almond milk if needed.

2 Add the banana and blend until smooth and creamy. Enjoy immediately.

BANANA ALMOND BUTTER SMOOTHIE

Serves: 2   **Prep Time:** 5 minutes   **Cook Time:** 0 minutes

This raw, vegan smoothie is a delicious way to start your day. Bananas and almonds are good sources of prebiotics.

1½ cups almond milk

¼ cup almond butter

Pinch sea salt

2 frozen bananas, cut into chunks

Combine all the ingredients in a blender and purée until smooth. Enjoy immediately.

DETOXIFYING GREEN SMOOTHIE

Serves: 2   **Prep Time:** 5 minutes   **Cook Time:** 0 minutes

This is my go-to green smoothie. Cilantro has natural chelating properties to detoxify your body from heavy metals and is antimicrobial. And I love the natural sweetness of the pineapple and the tartness of the citrus. For concentrated flavor, freeze the pineapple and add the frozen chunks at the end of the recipe.

2 cups fresh diced pineapple

1 lime, peeled

1 orange, peeled

1 small bunch fresh cilantro

4 cups dark leafy greens, such as kale or spinach

2 cups crushed ice

1 Place the pineapple, lime, and orange into a blender. Pulse a few times, adding water if needed to get things going. Purée until smooth.

2 Add the cilantro, greens, and ice and blend until very smooth. Enjoy immediately.

CHERRY CHEESECAKE SMOOTHIE

Serves: 2   **Prep Time:** 5 minutes   **Cook Time:** 0 minutes

This smoothie reminds me of the cherry cheesecakes my mom made for me on my birthday growing up. Cherries are a good source of prebiotics, and Greek yogurt is rich in probiotics.

1 cup full-fat Greek Yogurt (page 70)

1 cup non-fat milk

1 teaspoon vanilla extract

Pinch sea salt

2 cups frozen cherries

2 tablespoons toasted whole pecans

1 Combine all of the ingredients except the pecans in a blender and purée until very smooth, adding more milk if needed.

2 Add the pecans and pulse a few times until chopped into small pieces. Enjoy immediately.

TRIPLE BERRY SMOOTHIE

Serves: 2   **Prep Time:** 5 minutes   **Cook Time:** 0 minutes

All berries are rich sources of prebiotics, particularly the skins. For increased resistant starch, use a green banana. The smoothie is already sweet from the delicious berries.

1 cup hulled strawberries

1 cup blueberries

1 cup raspberries

¼ teaspoon vanilla extract

1 cup plain Greek Yogurt (page 70)

1 frozen banana, cut into chunks

Combine all of the ingredients in the order listed in the blender. Purée until smooth. Enjoy immediately.

MINT CHOCOLATE SMOOTHIE

Serves: 2   **Prep Time:** 5 minutes   **Cook Time:** 0 minutes

This smoothie is the Trojan horse of vegetable delivery methods. It's especially helpful for sneaking spinach into kids' meals ... not that I would know anything about that!

¼ cup fresh mint

2 cups fresh spinach

1 cup almond milk

2 tablespoons cocoa powder

2 frozen bananas, cut into chunks

Combine the mint, spinach, almond milk, and cocoa powder in a blender and purée until smooth. Add the frozen banana chunks and purée until thick and creamy. Enjoy immediately.

FERMENTED FOODS

PLAIN YOGURT

Yields: 4 quarts (16 cups)   **Prep Time:** 5 minutes, plus 4 to 8 hours inactive time   **Cook Time:** 5 minutes

Making your own yogurt is much easier than you might imagine and allows you to keep it pure and simple with no added sweeteners, fillers, or preservatives. If you're accustomed to eating processed yogurt with added sugar, homemade yogurt will taste a little different. But, it's so good for you and is loaded with probiotics to supplement a healthy microbiome.

1 gallon 2% or whole milk

1 cup plain yogurt with live-active cultures

1 Heat the milk in a large pot over medium–low heat until it reaches 200°F, not quite boiling. Allow it to cool to 115°F.

2 Remove 1 cup of the milk and stir it into the yogurt to temper it. Then stir the yogurt-milk mixture into the rest of the milk.

3 Cover the pot and place in a warm spot, such as a dehydrator or an oven at 110°F. Allow the yogurt to set for at least 4 hours without disturbing it. The longer you allow the yogurt to set, the tangier it will become. When it reaches the desired consistency and flavor, remove it and place in the refrigerator.

HONEY VANILLA YOGURT

Yields: 1 quart (4 cups)   **Prep Time:** 5 minutes   **Cook Time:** 0 minutes

This is the yogurt I grew up with. My mom always purchased plain yogurt but allowed us to stir in honey and vanilla to suit our young palates. Raw honey is a good source of probiotics. However, no variety of honey should be served to infants under one year old.

1 quart (4 cups) Plain Yogurt (page 68)

1 teaspoon vanilla extract

¼ cup raw honey, warmed slightly

Prepare the plain yogurt. Before placing in the refrigerator, stir in the vanilla and honey.

GREEK YOGURT

Yield: 1 to 1½ quarts (4 to 6 cups)   **Prep Time:** 5 minutes plus several hours inactive time   **Cook Time:** 0 minutes

You can easily make Greek yogurt from plain yogurt by straining it through several layers of cheesecloth. This removes some of the whey, which you can save for use in smoothies. Icelandic yogurt, called skyr, is similar, but uses non-fat milk in the yogurt-making process and is strained until it's thick enough to stand a spoon in it. Both Greek and Icelandic yogurts contain more protein per cup than unstrained yogurt.

2 quarts (8 cups) Plain Yogurt
(page 68)

1 Line a colander with several layers of cheesecloth and set the colander over a bowl.

2 Pour the yogurt into the colander and place in the refrigerator for several hours until it reaches the desired consistency. Discard the liquid or save it for another use, such as blending into smoothies or using in baking.

KEFIR

Yields: 1 cup   **Prep Time:** 5 minutes plus 24 hours inactive time
Cook Time: 0 minutes

Like yogurt, kefir (*kah-FEAR*) is fermented milk abounding in beneficial probiotics. Think of it like a sour, barely fizzy, drinkable yogurt. However, kefir uses a starter culture called kefir "grains" and does not require heating the milk first. Kefir grains can be purchased online or in a health food store and can be used again and again indefinitely if properly cared for by placing them in fresh milk to ferment a new batch or by placing in fresh milk and refrigerating. You can use 2% milk, but do not use shelf-stable milk.

1 teaspoon kefir grains   1 cup full-fat milk

1   Place the kefir grains in a glass jar. Pour in the milk. Cover lightly with cheesecloth or parchment paper, but do not screw on a metal lid.

2   Allow the milk to ferment for 24 hours at room temperature, at least 60°F but not more than 90°F. The kefir is ready when it is tangy and thick.

3   Before serving or storing, pour the liquid through a fine-mesh sieve to remove the kefir grains.

SPICY QUICK PICKLES

Yield: 1 quart   **Prep Time:** 10 minutes   **Cook Time:** 0 minutes

I loved pickles long before I became pregnant, but it was certainly a good excuse to indulge. These easy quick pickles resemble those that you find in the refrigerated section of the market, not the shelf-stable varieties.

1½ pounds Kirby cucumbers

1 tablespoon sea salt

1 tablespoon coriander seeds

2 garlic cloves, smashed

1 teaspoon red chile flakes

½ cup white wine vinegar

2 fresh dill sprigs, roughly chopped

1 Slice the cucumbers in ¼-inch-thick rounds.

2 In a 1-quart mason jar, combine the salt, coriander seeds, garlic cloves, and red chile flakes. Add the vinegar and stir to combine.

3 Add the sliced cucumbers and dill and seal the jar. Give it a good shake to fully coat the cucumber slices in the brine. Place the jar in the refrigerator and shake it again every 1 to 2 hours. Eventually, the cucumbers will release their liquid and the water level will rise.

4 The pickles are technically ready whenever you want to eat them, but they're best if you leave them to rest for several hours.

PRESERVED LEMONS

Serves: 2 to 4   **Prep Time:** 10 minutes   **Cook Time:** 1 to 2 minutes

Probiotics never tasted so good! Think salty, sweet lemon pickles. I like to keep a small batch in my refrigerator for adding to risotto, making a tangy harissa, and even adding to salad dressing.

1 teaspoon coriander seeds

1 teaspoon fennel seeds

2 lemons, scrubbed

¼ cup sea salt

1 teaspoon black peppercorns

1 In a small, dry skillet, toast the coriander and fennel seed over medium heat until fragrant, 1 to 2 minutes.

2 Cut the lemons into wedges lengthwise.

3 Add 1 tablespoon of the salt and about a third of the coriander, fennel, and peppercorns to a clean half-pint mason jar.

4 Squeeze the juice from two of the lemon wedges into the jar and stir. Stuff the lemon rinds down into the salt and juice.

5 Add another tablespoon of salt and a third of the spices. Squeeze the juice from another two lemon quarters into the jar and then add the rinds. Repeat until the jar is full and the lemon rinds are fully submerged in juice. Finish with the salt and spices. If your lemons are large, you may end up using all of the juice but not having room for the remaining two lemon rinds. Make sure the lemon rinds are covered with liquid. You may need to add the juice from another lemon.

6 Cover with a clean lid and place in a cool dark place for at least 5 days or up to 2 weeks before placing in the refrigerator.

SMALL-BATCH SAUERKRAUT

Yields: ½ pint (1 cup)   Prep Time: 5 minutes   Cook Time: 0 minutes

As I prepared to make my first batch of sauerkraut, I asked my husband, Rich, if he liked it. He reminded me that he had grown up in Germany. Enough said. What surprised me the most about my first batch was how sweet it smelled. I anticipated something a little more acerbic and, well, sour. What a pleasant surprise!

2 cups finely shredded Savoy cabbage   1 teaspoon sea salt

1 In a clean bowl, combine the cabbage and salt. Massage the cabbage with perfectly clean hands for a few minutes, until it softens and releases some of its liquid.

2 Place the cabbage into a clean half-pint jar, pressing down to make it fit. Top the cabbage with a small round of parchment paper and then press down with a heavy, slender object, such as a pestle from a mortar and pestle. Store the jar in a cool, dark place.

3 For the first 24 hours, pour off any excess liquid that rises above the parchment.

4 Taste the sauerkraut after 3 days. Allow it to continue fermenting for up to 1 week, or cover with a lid and store in the refrigerator.

SAUERKRAUT WITH JUNIPER AND CARAWAY

Yields: 1 pint (2 cups)   **Prep Time:** 5 minutes
Cook Time: 0 minutes

Caraway seeds are a classic addition to sauerkraut and give it an authentic taste. They also have antimicrobial properties.

1 head Savoy cabbage, finely shredded

2 teaspoons sea salt

1 teaspoon juniper berries

1 teaspoon caraway seeds

1 In a clean, large bowl, combine the cabbage and salt. Massage the cabbage with perfectly clean hands for a few minutes, until it softens and releases some of its liquid.

2 Place the cabbage, juniper berries, and caraway seeds into a clean pint jar, pressing down to make it fit. Top the cabbage with a small round of parchment paper and then press down with a heavy, slender object, such as a pestle from a mortar and pestle. Store the jar in a cool, dark place.

3 For the first 24 hours, pour off any excess liquid that rises above the parchment.

4 Taste the sauerkraut after 3 days. Allow it to continue fermenting for up to 1 week, or cover and store in the refrigerator.

KIMCHI

Yields: 2 quarts (8 cups)   **Prep Time:** 10 minutes
Cook Time: 0 minutes

Kimchi is a traditional Korean side dish that's delicious alongside a steaming bowl of pho. My first exposure to kimchi was in college, when I was regaled with stories of how the sophomore guys had smeared kimchi all along the halls of the freshmen girls' dorm just moments before they all left for the Christmas holiday. I can only imagine the smell! Whatever your intended use, plan to make the kimchi at least a week before you want to use it.

1 head Napa cabbage

2 tablespoons sea salt

2 green onions (green and white parts) cut into 1-inch segments

1 tablespoon fish sauce

2 tablespoons ground Korean red pepper (gochugaru)

¼ cup rice vinegar

1 tablespoon minced fresh ginger

4 garlic cloves, minced

1 Cut the cabbage head in quarters and remove the core. Slice each quarter into 2-inch strips. Place it in a very clean, large bowl. Sprinkle with the sea salt and massage the cabbage with clean hands until it begins to feel soft and releases its liquid, about 5 to 10 minutes. Add more salt as desired.

2 Add the green onions to the cabbage and toss to combine.

3 In a mortar and pestle, combine all of the remaining ingredients to make a paste. Pour the paste over the cabbage and onions and stir until thoroughly coated.

4 Place the cabbage mixture into a clean, 2-quart mason jar, pressing down to make it fit. Top the cabbage with a heavy object, such as a clean jar filled with water. Do not seal, or the gasses will not be able to escape. Store the jar in a cool, dark place.

5 Taste the kimchi after 1 week. Allow it to continue fermenting for up to 2 weeks, or cover and store in the refrigerator.

BASIC KOMBUCHA

Yields: 1 gallon   **Prep Time:** 30 minutes, plus 6 to 7 days inactive time   **Cook Time:** 5 minutes

I was pretty late to the kombucha party, but when I finally discovered how delicious it is and experienced the immediate soothing effects, I was hooked. It became an everyday habit—and an expensive one! Although home-brewing kombucha is intimidating at first, it is surprisingly easy and makes the daily drink far more economical. For your first batch, order the SCOBY online at Cultures for Health or request one from a friend who brews kombucha. The starter tea can be from a previous batch of kombucha from a friend or the SCOBY soaking liquid. However, commercial kombucha isn't a good starter.

1 gallon water
1 cup sugar
8 black tea bags

½ cup starter tea
1 SCOBY

1   Bring the water to a boil and then remove from the heat. Stir in the sugar until dissolved. Add the tea bags and allow it to steep until the tea is completely cool. Remove the tea bags.

2   Stir in the starter tea.

3   Pour the brew into a clean glass jar. Carefully place the SCOBY on the surface of the liquid.

4   Cover the jar with a coffee filter or paper towel and tighten with a rubber band. You want air to circulate freely but no pests or dust to enter.

5   Place the jar in a warm place out of direct sunlight, such as a pantry or laundry room, away from drafts.

6   Allow the brew to rest for at least 5 days. Taste with a straw. When the kombucha reaches the desired balance of sweet and sour, it is ready to bottle. Warmer climates at least 75°F will ferment the kombucha more quickly than cooler kitchen environments.

7   If you're making the basic kombucha, divide it between individual glass jars, leaving at least 1 inch of head room in each. Top with plastic lids. Alternatively, add your chosen flavoring before filling the bottles with kombucha.

8 After bottling, reuse the SCOBY and 1 cup of the kombucha to start your next batch.

9 Return the jars to the pantry or a cupboard for 24 to 48 hours to allow them to carbonate. You may want to open one jar on your first batch to test for carbonation.

10 Carefully store the jars in the refrigerator and avoid jostling or shaking them. Enjoy when chilled.

LEMON GINGER KOMBUCHA

Yields: 1 gallon   **Prep Time:** 5 minutes, plus 24 to 48 hours inactive time   **Cook Time:** 0 minutes

Begin with the Basic Kombucha and add your own flavors for a delicious, healthy twist. To make the ginger juice, grate about 2 to 3 tablespoons of fresh ginger over a Microplane grater and then squeeze it using a coffee filter or nut milk bag.

1 tablespoon ginger juice

2 tablespoons lemon juice

2 tablespoons raw honey

1 recipe Basic Kombucha (page 77)

1 Whisk together the ginger juice, lemon juice, and honey. Divide the sweetened juice between individual glass bottles.

2 Divide the kombucha between the bottles, leaving at least 1 inch of head room in each. Top with plastic lids.

3 Return the jars to a dark corner for 24 to 48 hours to allow them to carbonate. You may want to open one jar on your first batch to test for carbonation.

4 Carefully store the jars in the refrigerator and avoid jostling or shaking them.

BERRY BLISS KOMBUCHA

Yields: 1 gallon   **Prep Time:** 5 minutes, plus 24 to 48 hours inactive time   **Cook Time:** 0 minutes

Use whatever berries are in season, or use frozen defrosted berries, which easily release their liquid. It is fine to mash and use the whole fruit to make flavored kombucha, but I prefer a smoother texture, so I just use the fruit juice.

1 pint blackberries

1 pint strawberries

1 teaspoon lemon juice

1 recipe Basic Kombucha (page 77)

1 Combine the blackberries, strawberries, and lemon juice in a blender. Press the juices through a strainer. Divide the juice between individual glass bottles.

2 Divide the kombucha between the bottles, leaving at least 1 inch of head room in each. Top with plastic lids.

3 Return the jars to a dark corner for 24 to 48 hours to allow them to carbonate. You may want to open one jar on your first batch to test for carbonation.

4 Carefully store the jars in the refrigerator and avoid jostling or shaking them.

VANILLA PEACH KOMBUCHA

Yields: 1 gallon   **Prep Time:** 5 minutes, plus 24 to 48 hours inactive time   **Cook Time:** 0 minutes

Vanilla beans can be pretty expensive, but I like to purchase them from the Mexican food aisle of my supermarket, where the beans are sold individually for a fraction of the cost in the spice aisle.

2 very ripe peaches, pitted

1 split vanilla bean

1 recipe Basic Kombucha (page 77)

1 Purée the peaches in a blender. Press the juices through a strainer. Divide the juice between individual glass bottles. Using a sharp pair of kitchen shears, snip the vanilla bean into pieces so that one is in each bottle.

2 Divide the kombucha between the bottles, leaving at least 1 inch of head room in each. Top with plastic lids.

3 Return the jars to a dark corner for 24 to 48 hours to allow them to carbonate. You may want to open one jar on your first batch to test for carbonation.

4 Carefully store the jars in the refrigerator and avoid jostling or shaking them.

MANGO CITRUS KOMBUCHA

Yields: 1 gallon   **Prep Time:** 5 minutes, plus 24 to 48 hours inactive time   **Cook Time:** 0 minutes

This kombucha recipe is bright, tangy, and a little sweeter than other kombucha flavors.

1 cup cubed mango

Zest and juice of 1 orange

Zest and juice of 1 lime

1 recipe Basic Kombucha (page 77)

1 Purée the mango in a blender with the orange and lime zest and juices. Press the mixture through a strainer; it will not be clear. Divide the juice between individual glass bottles.

2 Divide the kombucha between the bottles, leaving at least 1 inch of head room in each. Top with plastic lids.

3 Return the jars to a dark corner for 24 to 48 hours to allow them to carbonate. You may want to open one jar on your first batch to test for carbonation.

4 Carefully store the jars in the refrigerator and avoid jostling or shaking them.

LAVENDER SAGE KOMBUCHA

Yields: 1 gallon   **Prep Time:** 5 minutes, plus 24 to 48 hours inactive time   **Cook Time:** 2 minutes

Lavender and sage bring a beautiful aroma and complex flavor to this lightly sweetened kombucha.

1 cup water

2 tablespoons lavender

2 fresh sage sprigs

2 tablespoons raw honey

1 recipe Basic Kombucha (page 77)

1 Bring the water to a simmer in a small sauce pan with the lavender and sage for 2 minutes. Muddle them with a wooden spoon to release their oils. Remove the pan from the heat and allow the "tea" to steep for 30 minutes. Strain the mixture and stir in the honey.

2 Divide the lavender "tea" between individual glass bottles.

3 Divide the kombucha between the bottles, leaving at least 1 inch of head room in each. Top with plastic lids.

4 Return the jars to a dark corner for 24 to 48 hours to allow them to carbonate. You may want to open one jar on your first batch to test for carbonation.

5 Carefully store the jars in the refrigerator and avoid jostling or shaking them.

7

VEGETARIAN ENTRÉES

Lemony Quinoa and Kale Bliss Bowl

Fresh Basil and Tomato Pasta with Olive Oil

Loaded Sweet Potatoes with Barbecue Sauce

Vegan Bean and Rice Burritos

Baja Bowls with Mole

Indian Coconut Curry with Spinach and Sweet Potatoes

Chickpea and Yogurt Curry with Cardamom

Korean Rice Bowls

Broccoli Tofu Stir-Fry

Buckwheat Noodle and Edamame Stir-Fry

Spaghetti Squash Bowls with Mushroom Primavera

Goat Cheese Polenta with Roasted Fennel and Dates

LEMONY QUINOA AND KALE BLISS BOWL

Serves: 2 **Prep Time:** 10 minutes **Cook Time:** 20 minutes

I love the rich color and firm texture of red quinoa, but use whatever you have available. The preserved lemons add a healthy dose of probiotics coupled with the prebiotics in the quinoa, kale, and garlic.

1 cup red quinoa

2 cups vegetable broth or water

¼ Preserved Lemon (page 73), minced

¼ cup minced fresh flat-leaf parsley

1 plum tomato, seeded and diced

1 bunch kale, ribs removed

2 garlic cloves, minced, divided

2 to 3 tablespoons extra-virgin olive oil

Pinch sea salt

1 (15-ounce) can chickpeas, rinsed and drained

1 teaspoon smoked paprika

1 teaspoon ground cumin

1 tablespoon red wine vinegar

¼ cup pine nuts, toasted, roughly chopped

1 Bring the quinoa and broth to a simmer in a medium pot over medium–low heat. Cover and cook until tender, about 20 minutes

2 Add the preserved lemon, parsley, and tomato to the quinoa and fluff with a fork.

3 Chop the kale into bite-size pieces. In a large bowl, combine the kale, half of the garlic, olive oil, and the pinch of sea salt. Massage the olive oil into the kale leaves, squeezing it with your hands until it is slightly softened. You may not need to use all of the olive oil to thoroughly coat all of the leaves.

4 In a separate bowl, combine the chickpeas, the remaining half of the garlic, and the paprika, cumin, and vinegar. Toss to coat.

5 Divide the quinoa between four bowls. Top with kale, chickpeas, and pine nuts.

FRESH BASIL AND TOMATO PASTA WITH OLIVE OIL

Serves: 4   **Prep Time:** 10 minutes, plus 15 minutes inactive time
Cook Time: 10 minutes

Use the best quality extra-virgin olive oil you can find and the freshest tomatoes in season. This is best in late summer, and it's perfect for doubling and feeding a crowd. I like to use quinoa noodles or fresh gluten-free pasta, but use whatever suits your taste.

½ cup extra-virgin olive oil

2 pounds assorted heirloom tomatoes, cut into bite-size pieces

2 cups hand-torn fresh basil

4 garlic cloves, minced

Sea salt

Freshly ground black pepper

16 ounces quinoa or corn spaghetti noodles

8 ounces fresh mozzarella, torn into bite-size pieces

1   Combine the olive oil, tomatoes, basil, and garlic in a large serving bowl. Season with salt and pepper. Allow to sit for at least 15 minutes to bring the flavors together.

2   Meanwhile, bring a large pot of salted water to a boil over medium heat. Cook the pasta according to the package directions. Drain thoroughly.

3   Add the pasta to the serving dish along with the mozzarella. Give everything a good toss and allow to rest for a few minutes before serving to gently warm the olive oil and slightly melt the mozzarella.

LOADED SWEET POTATOES WITH BARBECUE SAUCE

Serves: 2 to 4   **Prep Time:** 15 minutes   **Cook Time:** 45 minutes

This might be my absolute favorite recipe in this book. It shows up on my weekly menu again and again. The unpeeled sweet potatoes and cabbage are loaded with prebiotics and the tempeh is filled with probiotics for a symbiotic meal that tastes amazing!

2 to 3 sweet potatoes, unpeeled

3 tablespoons extra-virgin olive oil, divided

Sea salt

1 (8-ounce) package tempeh

1 cup Barbecue Sauce (page 123) or store-bought sauce

2 tablespoons mayonnaise

2 tablespoons lime juice

1 teaspoon ground cumin

4 cups shredded Savoy cabbage

1 Preheat the oven to 400°F.

2 Slice the sweet potatoes lengthwise in ¼-inch-thick pieces. Place them on a sheet pan. Drizzle with 2 tablespoons of the oil and toss gently to coat. Season with salt.

3 Roast uncovered for 40 minutes, or until the bottoms are browned and the tops are shrunken.

4 Meanwhile, heat the remaining tablespoon of oil in a large skillet. Crumble the tempeh and sauté over medium heat until browned, 3 to 4 minutes. Add the barbecue sauce and cook until just heated through.

5 In a large bowl, whisk together the mayonnaise, lime juice, and cumin. Add the cabbage and toss to coat thoroughly.

6 To serve, place the sweet potatoes into individual bowls. Top with a generous scoop of the tempeh and then the cabbage. Serve immediately.

VEGAN BEAN AND RICE BURRITOS

Serves: 4   **Prep Time:** 20 minutes   **Cook Time:** 0 minutes

These carbohydrate-loaded burritos are energizing and packed with prebiotics to feed your microbiome.

1 cup cooked brown rice

1 cup refried beans

1 cup corn kernels

1 cup canned fire-roasted diced tomatoes, drained

½ red onion, diced

1 red bell pepper, cored and diced

1 cup roughly chopped fresh cilantro

4 large gluten-free tortillas

1 cup prepared guacamole, or 2 whole avocados, diced

4 tablespoons hot sauce, such as Cholula

1 In a large bowl, combine the rice, beans, corn, tomatoes, onion, bell pepper, and cilantro.

2 Divide the mixture between the four tortillas. Top each with ¼ cup of guacamole and 1 tablespoon of hot sauce.

BAJA BOWLS WITH MOLE

Serves: 4   **Prep Time:** 15 minutes   **Cook Time:** 50 minutes

Long before fresh Mexican food was a common fast food offering, a small counter-service restaurant chain in Portland, Oregon, offered these rice and bean bowls. I was a teenager when I first tried it, and fell in love with the combination of rice and beans smothered in tangy pico de gallo, guacamole, and smoky mole.

1 cup long-grain brown rice

2 cups water

Sea salt

1 (15-ounce) can kidney beans, rinsed and drained

1 teaspoon ground cumin

1 teaspoon smoked paprika

¼ teaspoon cayenne pepper

1 garlic clove, minced

1 cup corn kernels

1 cup Guacamole (page 112)

1 cup Pico de Gallo (page 112)

1 cup Mole (page 113)

Lime wedges, for serving

1 Bring the rice and water to a simmer with a generous pinch of sea salt in a pot. Cover and cook on low for 45 minutes, or until al dente.

2 In a small sauce pan, combine the kidney beans, cumin, paprika, cayenne, and garlic. Cook until heated through, about 5 minutes.

3 Divide the rice and beans between 4 bowls. Top with the corn kernels, guacamole, and pico de gallo, and drizzle with mole. Serve with lime wedges.

INDIAN COCONUT CURRY WITH SPINACH AND SWEET POTATOES

Serves: 2 to 4   **Prep Time:** 10 minutes
Cook Time: 15 to 20 minutes

I adore this combination of spices, adapted from a recipe in *Gourmet* magazine. If you can't find fresh curry leaves, simply omit them, but do not try to substitute curry powder; it is an entirely different ingredient. Serve over cooked rice.

1 tablespoon coriander seeds

1 tablespoon cumin seeds

6 fresh curry leaves (optional)

¼ teaspoon red chile flakes

2 tablespoons extra-virgin olive oil

1 yellow onion, halved and thinly sliced

3 garlic cloves, minced

1 tablespoon lime juice

1 teaspoon tomato paste

½ teaspoon ground turmeric

1 (15-ounce) can full-fat coconut milk

2 cups low-sodium vegetable broth

2 sweet potatoes, peeled and diced

4 cups roughly chopped fresh spinach

1 lime, cut into wedges for serving

Sea salt

1 Toast the coriander seeds, cumin seeds, curry leaves, and red chile flakes in a dry skillet over medium heat until fragrant, 1 to 2 minutes.

2 Remove the pan from the heat and transfer the spices to a mortar and pestle or spice grinder. Pulverize into a fine powder.

3 In a large pot, heat the olive oil over medium heat. Cook the onion and garlic with a generous pinch of sea salt for 5 minutes.

4 Add the ground spices, lime juice, tomato paste, turmeric, coconut milk, and vegetable broth. Bring to a simmer and add the sweet potatoes. Cover and cook for 15 to 20 minutes, until the sweet potato is tender. Season with salt, then stir in the spinach. Serve with lime wedges.

CHICKPEA AND YOGURT CURRY WITH CARDAMOM

Serves: 2   **Prep Time:** 10 minutes   **Cook Time:** 15 minutes

This fragrant curry is loaded with prebiotics and probiotics from the plain yogurt. Make sure to remove the pan from the heat to allow it to cool slightly before stirring in the yogurt to retain its probiotic benefits.

1 tablespoon cumin seeds

2 teaspoons coriander seeds

½ teaspoon ground cinnamon

¼ teaspoon ground cardamom

1 teaspoon garam masala

2 tablespoons coconut oil

1 yellow onion, diced

2 tablespoons minced fresh ginger

4 garlic cloves, minced

2 ripe tomatoes, seeded and diced

2 cups thinly sliced spinach

2 (15-ounce) cans chickpeas, rinsed and drained

1 cup Plain Yogurt (page 68)

¼ cup roughly chopped fresh cilantro

1 Toast the cumin and coriander seeds in a large, dry skillet over medium heat for 1 to 2 minutes, until fragrant. Transfer them to a spice grinder or mortar and pestle. Pulverize until finely ground. Add the cinnamon, cardamom, and garam masala and set aside.

2 In the same skillet, add the coconut oil and cook the onion over medium heat until slightly softened, 5 minutes. Add the ginger and garlic and cook for another 1 to 2 minutes, until fragrant. Add the ground spices, tomatoes, and spinach. Stir until the spinach is wilted and giving up some of its liquid, about 1 minute.

3 Stir in the chickpeas and cook for 1 to 2 minutes more.

4 Remove the pan from the heat and stir in the yogurt. Garnish with fresh cilantro.

KOREAN RICE BOWLS

Serves: 4   **Prep Time:** 15 minutes   **Cook Time:** 50 minutes

The ingredient list is long here, but these bowls come together quickly if you prep the ingredients ahead of time. They're really amazing if you make your own kimchi, but store-bought will work just as well.

1½ cups brown basmati rice

3 cups water

1 tablespoon toasted sesame oil

2 cups thinly sliced shiitake mushrooms

1 tablespoon minced garlic

1 bunch spinach

1 cup shredded carrots

1 cup shredded red cabbage

4 green onions (green and white parts) thinly sliced on a bias

1 cup bean sprouts

1 cup Kimchi (page 76)

2 tablespoons canola oil

4 eggs

Gochujang, for serving

Sea salt

Freshly ground pepper

1 Bring the rice and water to a simmer with a generous pinch of sea salt in a pot. Cover and cook on low for 45 minutes, or until al dente.

2 When the rice is nearly done, heat the sesame oil over medium heat in a large skillet. Sauté the mushrooms for 4 to 5 minutes, until browned. Add the garlic and cook for 30 seconds. Add the spinach and cook until it is just barely wilted. Remove from the heat. Season with salt and pepper.

3 Divide the cooked rice between 4 bowls. Top with the sautéed mushrooms and spinach. Divide the carrots, cabbage, onions, bean sprouts, and kimchi between the bowls.

4 Heat a large skillet over medium heat. When it is hot, add the canola oil. Tilt the pan to coat. Fry the eggs until the whites are set and the yolks are still runny. Season with salt and pepper.

5 Set one egg atop each of the rice bowls. Serve with gochujang.

BROCCOLI TOFU STIR-FRY

Serves: 2 to 4   **Prep Time:** 10 minutes   **Cook Time:** 45 minutes

Make takeout at home with this simple broccoli and tofu stir-fry. Feel free to use a store-bought peanut sauce if you want, or make healthy Peanut Sauce (page 121) from scratch.

1½ cups long-grain brown rice

3 cups water

Sea salt

2 tablespoons toasted sesame oil

1 (16-ounce) block extra-firm tofu

1 head broccoli, cut into florets

1 yellow onion, halved and thinly sliced

1 recipe Peanut Sauce (page 121)

Juice of 1 lime, plus 1 lime, cut into wedges

½ cup roughly chopped fresh cilantro

1   Bring the rice and water to a simmer with a pinch of sea salt over medium heat. Cover, reduce the heat to low, and cook until tender, about 45 minutes.

2   Meanwhile, slice the tofu in half horizontally. Fold several pieces of paper towels and set the tofu on them. Fold several additional paper towels and set them on top of the tofu. Top with a cutting board and then weigh it down with a few heavy kitchen objects. Allow the tofu to release moisture for at least 30 minutes. Remove the pressed tofu.

3   Heat the sesame oil in a large skillet over medium–high heat. Sear the tofu for about 5 minutes, until a golden brown crust forms. Flip and cook on the other side for another 5 minutes. Remove the tofu to a cutting board. When it is cool enough to handle, slice it into 1-inch cubes.

4   Cook the broccoli and onion in the same skillet for 5 to 10 minutes, until bright green and slightly tender.

5   Reduce the heat to low and add the tofu, peanut sauce, and lime juice. Cook for 2 to 3 more minutes. Serve the cooked tofu and broccoli over the cooked rice and garnish with the lime wedges and cilantro.

BUCKWHEAT NOODLE AND EDAMAME STIR-FRY

Serves: 2 to 4   **Prep Time:** 10 minutes   **Cook Time:** 15 minutes

Despite its name, buckwheat is unrelated to wheat. However, if you are gluten-sensitive or allergic to wheat, make sure to look for 100 percent buckwheat noodles that are certified gluten-free. To save time, prepare the noodles and sauce and chop all of the vegetables ahead of time. You can have dinner on the table in a mere 10 minutes!

1 (8-ounce) package buckwheat noodles

¼ cup low-sodium, gluten-free soy sauce

2 tablespoons lime juice

1 tablespoon raw honey

1 tablespoon minced ginger

1 teaspoon minced garlic

1 shallot, minced

2 tablespoons toasted sesame oil

1 yellow onion, halved and thinly sliced

2 carrots, cut into matchsticks

2 cups snow peas, strings removed

1 cup blanched, shelled edamame

½ cup roughly chopped fresh cilantro

1 Cook the buckwheat noodles according to package directions. Rinse with cool water, drain, and set aside.

2 To make the sauce, combine the soy sauce, lime juice, honey, ginger, garlic, and shallot in a glass jar. Shake to combine. Set aside.

3 Heat the sesame oil in a large skillet or wok over medium-high heat. Sauté the onion for 2 to 3 minutes. Add the carrots and snow peas and sauté for another 2 to 3 minutes.

4 Add the edamame and noodles and cook until the noodles are heated through, about 2 minutes.

5 Add the sauce and cook for another minute.

6 To serve, divide the mixture between plates or bowls and top with the cilantro.

SPAGHETTI SQUASH BOWLS WITH MUSHROOM PRIMAVERA

Serves: 2   **Prep Time:** 10 minutes   **Cook Time:** 45 minutes

As its name suggests, the flesh of spaghetti squash forms thin noodles that can be raked with a fork to form a loose pile of pasta. Top it with a hearty mushroom marinara sauce for a healthy, filling vegetarian meal.

2 spaghetti squash

1 tablespoon extra-virgin olive oil

1 yellow onion, halved and thinly sliced

2 tablespoons salted butter

2 cups sliced cremini mushrooms

2 garlic cloves, minced

Pinch red chile flakes

1 teaspoon Italian herb blend

1 (15-ounce) can plum tomatoes

1 (15-ounce) can tomato sauce

1 cup roughly chopped fresh basil

½ cup finely grated Parmesan cheese

Sea salt

Freshly ground black pepper

1 Preheat the oven to 400°F.

2 Cut the spaghetti squash in half lengthwise and scoop out the seeds. Place the squash cut-side down in a casserole dish. Bake for 30 to 40 minutes, until the flesh is softened but not shriveled.

3 Meanwhile, heat the olive oil in a large skillet over medium heat. Season the onions with a pinch of sea salt and cook for 10 minutes until golden and soft. Push them to the sides of the pan.

4 Melt 1 to 2 teaspoons of the butter in the center of the skillet. Brown the mushrooms on each side for 1 to 2 minutes. You should do this in batches to not overcrowd the pan. Push the browned mushrooms to the side and add more butter and mushrooms until all are browned.

5 Add the garlic and red chile flakes to the pan and cook for another 30 seconds. Add the Italian herb blend, tomatoes, and tomato sauce. Simmer for 15 to 20 minutes, or until the spaghetti squash are done.

6 Stir in the basil. Adjust the seasoning to taste with salt and pepper.

7 When the spaghetti squash are finished baking, turn them flesh-side up and run a fork through the flesh to produce long, thin strands. Top each serving with a generous scoop of marinara sauce and a sprinkle of fresh Parmesan.

GOAT CHEESE POLENTA WITH ROASTED FENNEL AND DATES

Serves: 4   **Prep Time:** 5 minutes   **Cook Time:** 45 minutes

Polenta is often made with Parmesan cheese. I love goat cheese in this version because it's a good source of probiotics and provides a tangy creaminess. Microgreens are packed with nutrients and provide textural contrast, but you could also use tender spring greens if you wish.

2 fennel bulbs, cored and cut into eighths

¼ cup extra-virgin olive oil

Sea salt

Freshly ground black pepper

8 Medjool dates, pitted and thinly sliced

3 cups water

½ teaspoon sea salt

1 scant cup yellow cornmeal

4 ounces goat cheese, crumbled

2 cups microgreens

1   Preheat the oven to 375°F.

2   Spread the fennel on a rimmed baking sheet and drizzle with the olive oil. Toss to coat thoroughly. Season with salt and pepper. Roast uncovered for 45 minutes, or until tender and caramelized. During the last 5 minutes of cooking, add the dates to the pan and stir together with the fennel to coat in the olive oil.

3   Meanwhile, bring the water and sea salt to a gentle simmer over medium heat. Slowly pour in the cornmeal, stirring constantly. Reduce the heat to low and cook for 15 minutes. During the last few minutes of cooking, stir in the goat cheese.

4   Divide the polenta between serving plates. Top with the roasted fennel and dates and a handful of microgreens.

8

MEAT, POULTRY, & FISH

Pan-Seared Scallops over Polenta

Miso-Glazed Salmon

Salmon Cakes and Potato Skins

Cashew Chicken and Mango Stir-Fry

Pistachio-Crusted Chicken Breast with Yogurt Sauce

Roasted Chicken and Sweet Potatoes with Mole

Chicken, Cauliflower, and Raisins over Quinoa

Chicken Thighs with Smashed Potatoes

Flank Steak Tacos with Chimichurri

Grilled Lamb Chops with Pistachio Mint Pesto

PAN-SEARED SCALLOPS OVER POLENTA

Serves: 4   **Prep Time:** 5 minutes   **Cook Time:** 20 minutes

Polenta is made from ground corn and is a rich source of resistant starch. Ghee is clarified butter. It can be used to cook at higher heat because it contains no milk solids, which also makes it more easily digestible for people who are sensitive to dairy.

3 cups water

½ teaspoon sea salt

1 scant cup yellow cornmeal

2 tablespoons ghee

1 pound large sea scallops

Sea salt

Freshly ground black pepper

2 tablespoons minced fresh flat-leaf parsley

Juice of 1 lemon

1   Bring the water and sea salt to a gentle simmer over medium heat. Slowly pour in the cornmeal, stirring constantly. Reduce the heat to low and cook for 15 minutes.

2   Meanwhile, heat the ghee in a large skillet over medium-high heat.

3   Pat the scallops dry with paper towels and season with salt and pepper. Sear on each side for 3 to 4 minutes, basting with the ghee and pan juices. Flip and cook for 3 to 4 minutes on the other side until cooked through.

4   Divide the polenta between serving plates. Top each with scallops and fresh parsley. Shower with lemon juice.

MISO-GLAZED SALMON

Serves: 4   **Prep Time:** 5 minutes   **Cook Time:** 7 minutes

The umami flavors and probiotic benefits of miso are a delicious and healthy complement to salmon. Especially when it is wild caught, salmon is rich in gut-nourishing omega-3 fatty acids. Serve with Sweet Potato Fries (page 178).

1 pound salmon fillet

1 tablespoon toasted sesame oil

Sea salt

Freshly ground black pepper

2 tablespoons white miso paste

2 tablespoons gluten-free, low-sodium soy sauce

1 tablespoon rice vinegar

1 teaspoon raw honey

1 Preheat the broiler to high and place an oven rack about 5 inches from the heating element.

2 Coat the salmon flesh with the sesame oil and then season with salt and pepper.

3 Place the salmon skin-side down on a broiler pan and cook under the broiler for 5 minutes.

4 Meanwhile, whisk together the miso, soy sauce, vinegar, and honey.

5 Remove the salmon from the oven and examine the fish for its level of doneness. The interior flesh should be a darker shade of pink but easily flake with a fork when done.

6 Drizzle with the sauce and return to the oven for 1 to 2 more minutes.

SALMON CAKES AND POTATO SKINS

Serves: 2 to 4   **Prep Time:** 10 minutes   **Cook Time:** 1 hour 10 minutes

Potatoes, instead of bread crumbs, absorb excess moisture in these delicious salmon cakes. As a bonus, the potato skins make a yummy side dish. The prep time does seem long, but you can prepare the potatoes ahead of time and then assemble and cook at the last minute.

2 medium russet potatoes

1 egg, whisked

2 scallions, minced

1 (16-ounce) can wild salmon

4 tablespoons extra-virgin olive oil, divided

1 lemon, cut into wedges, for serving

2 cups arugula, for serving

Sea salt

Freshly ground black pepper

1   Preheat the oven to 400°F. Pierce the potatoes several times with a fork and place them directly on the oven rack. Bake for 45 minutes, until cooked through. Allow them to cool and then slice into quarters lengthwise.

2   Scoop out most of the potato flesh and put it into a large bowl. Add the egg and scallions and season generously with salt and pepper. Mix until thoroughly integrated. Add the salmon and stir until just combined. You want a few large chunks of salmon to remain.

3   Spread the potato skins on a rimmed baking sheet and brush with 2 tablespoons of the olive oil. Season with salt and pepper. Return to the oven for 15 minutes, or until gently browned and crisp.

4   Heat the remaining 2 tablespoons of oil in a large skillet. Form the salmon mixture into 6 patties and pan-fry for about 4 minutes, until browned and set. Flip carefully and cook on the other side until browned and heated through.

5   Serve with lemon wedges and a small handful of arugula.

CASHEW CHICKEN AND MANGO STIR-FRY

Serves: 4 **Prep Time:** 10 minutes **Cook Time:** 15 minutes

This quick stir-fry has a delicious balance of sweet, sour, salty, and savory flavors. The cashews, mangos, snap peas, and garlic all contain healthy prebiotics and the fish sauce and honey are brimming with probiotics. Serve alone or over steamed brown rice.

1 pound boneless, skinless chicken thighs, cut into 1-inch chunks

2 tablespoons coconut oil

Sea salt

Freshly ground black pepper

2 cups sugar snap peas, strings removed

1 teaspoon minced garlic

¼ teaspoon red chile flakes

¼ cup fish sauce

2 tablespoons lime juice

1 tablespoon raw honey

2 mangos, peeled, cored, and diced

1 cup roasted cashews

1 Season the chicken thighs with salt and pepper. Heat the coconut oil in a large skillet over medium–high heat. Brown the chicken on all sides until just cooked through, about 5 to 7 minutes. Transfer to a separate dish.

2 Place the sugar snap peas in the skillet and sauté for 5 minutes.

3 Lower the heat to medium. Add the garlic and red chile flakes and cook for about 30 seconds.

4 In a small bowl, whisk together the fish sauce, lime juice, and honey.

5 Return the chicken to the pan and add the fish sauce mixture. Cook until heated through, about 1 minute.

6 Add the mango and cashews, toss gently to combine, and remove from the heat.

PISTACHIO-CRUSTED CHICKEN BREAST WITH YOGURT SAUCE

Serves: 2   **Prep Time:** 10 minutes   **Cook Time:** 25 minutes

Pistachios make a crunchy coating for pan-fried chicken breasts and are a good source of resistant starch. Drizzle with the probiotic-rich yogurt sauce for a delicious symbiotic meal.

1 cup shelled pistachios

4 boneless, skinless chicken breasts

2 tablespoons canola oil

1 cup full-fat Plain Yogurt (page 68)

1 tablespoon lime juice

¼ teaspoon cayenne pepper

¼ teaspoon ground cumin

6 cups arugula

¼ cup mint leaves (optional)

Sea salt

Freshly ground black pepper

1 Preheat the oven to 375°F.

2 Grind the pistachios coarsely in a food processor. Season the chicken breasts on all sides with salt and pepper, and then dredge in the ground pistachios until well coated.

3 Heat the oil in a large, ovenproof skillet over medium-high heat. Brown the chicken on one side for 5 minutes, until golden. Flip the chicken and cook for another 5 minutes. Place the pan in the oven and cook for 15 minutes, or until the chicken is cooked through.

4 Meanwhile, in a small bowl, whisk together the yogurt, lime juice, cayenne, and cumin. Season to taste with salt and pepper.

5 Divide the arugula and mint leaves, if using, between serving plates. Top each with one piece of chicken and drizzle with the yogurt sauce.

ROASTED CHICKEN AND SWEET POTATOES WITH MOLE

Serves: 4   **Prep Time:** 10 minutes   **Cook Time:** 30 minutes

I love the flavors of roasted sweet potatoes and chicken smothered in a smoky mole sauce. Serve this on its own, over steamed brown rice, or as a filling for warmed corn tortillas.

4 boneless, skinless chicken breasts

2 large sweet potatoes, peeled and diced

2 tablespoons extra-virgin olive oil

Sea salt

Freshly ground black pepper

1 recipe Mole (page 113)

¼ cup green onions (green and white parts) thinly sliced

Corn tortillas, warmed, for serving

1 Preheat the oven to 400°F.

2 Spread the chicken and sweet potatoes out on a rimmed baking sheet and coat with the olive oil. Season with salt and pepper.

3 Roast uncovered until the chicken is cooked through and the sweet potatoes are gently browned, about 30 minutes.

4 Remove the chicken from the pan and cut into large chunks. Return it to the pan.

5 Pour the mole over the sweet potatoes and chicken, and give everything a good toss. Transfer to a serving dish and top with the green onions. Serve with warmed corn tortillas.

CHICKEN, CAULIFLOWER, AND RAISINS OVER QUINOA

Serves: 4   **Prep Time:** 10 minutes   **Cook Time:** 30 to 35 minutes

Cauliflower, quinoa, and raisins are rich sources of prebiotics. They also keep the meal filling without relying heavily on meat.

1 cup quinoa

2 cups Chicken Bone Broth (page 57)

2 tablespoons extra-virgin olive oil

2 chicken breasts, cut into 2-inch pieces

Sea salt

Freshly ground black pepper

1 head cauliflower, broken into florets

2 garlic cloves, minced

¼ cup raisins

¼ cup minced fresh flat-leaf parsley

Zest and juice of 1 lemon

1   Bring the quinoa and broth to a simmer over medium heat. Cover and cook on low for 15 to 20 minutes, or until all of the liquid is absorbed.

2   Heat the olive oil in a large skillet. Season the chicken on all sides with salt and pepper and fry until browned and just cooked through. Set it aside in a separate dish. Add the cauliflower to the pan, cover and cook until tender, about 10 minutes.

3   Add the garlic, raisins, and cooked chicken along with any accumulated juices to the pan. Cook until everything is heated through, another 1 to 2 minutes. Shower with the fresh parsley and lemon juice.

4   Fluff the quinoa with a fork and divide it among serving bowls. Top with the cauliflower and chicken.

CHICKEN THIGHS WITH SMASHED POTATOES

Serves: 2 to 4   **Prep Time:** 10 minutes   **Cook Time:** 45 minutes

There's something sublime about twice-baked potatoes. These get a generous dose of flavor from the prebiotic-rich olive and herb dressing.

1¼ pounds red-skinned potatoes

5 tablespoons extra-virgin olive oil, divided

4 bone-in, skin-on chicken thighs

Sea salt

Freshly ground black pepper

¼ cup minced fresh flat-leaf parsley

3 tablespoons minced kalamata olives

1 tablespoon red wine vinegar

1 teaspoon minced fresh thyme

1 shallot, minced

1 Preheat the oven to 375°F.

2 Spread the potatoes out onto a rimmed baking sheet and pierce each one with a fork. Roast for 30 minutes.

3 While the potatoes are cooking, heat 2 tablespoons of the olive oil in a large skillet. Season the chicken thighs liberally with salt and pepper. Cook skin-side down until brown and crisp, about 10 minutes. Flip to the other side and cook for another 10 minutes.

4 Remove the potatoes from the oven. Carefully smash each one with the flat side of a knife or a meat cleaver. Return them to the pan, brush with 2 tablespoons of the olive oil, and season with salt and pepper.

5 Add the chicken skin-side up to the pan and return to the oven for 15 minutes, or until the chicken is cooked through.

6 Meanwhile, combine the parsley, olives, vinegar, thyme, shallot and the remaining tablespoon of olive oil.

7 To serve, divide the potatoes and chicken between serving plates and top the potatoes with the olive mixture.

FLANK STEAK TACOS WITH CHIMICHURRI

Serves: 2 to 4   **Prep Time:** 5 minutes, plus 30 minutes to 8 hours inactive time   **Cook Time:** 10 minutes

Street tacos are one of my favorite summer foods, and I love using cabbage leaves instead of corn tortillas for a filling, low-carb meal.

1 pound flank steak

1 recipe Chimichurri (page 115)

8 corn tortillas or Savoy cabbage leaves

1 avocado, sliced

¼ cup diced red onion

1 Place the steak in a non-reactive dish and coat with 1 cup of the chimichurri. Allow to marinate for at least 30 minutes or up to 8 hours.

2 Preheat an outdoor grill or grill pan to medium-high heat.

3 Remove the steak from the marinade and pat dry. Place it on the grill for 5 minutes, flip, and cook for another 5 minutes, or until it reaches your desired level of doneness. Remove the meat to a cutting board to rest for 5 minutes.

4 Using a sharp knife, slice the meat on a bias into very thin strips. Divide them between the tortillas or cabbage leaves and top with avocado, red onion, and a drizzle of the remaining chimichurri.

GRILLED LAMB CHOPS WITH PISTACHIO MINT PESTO

Serves: 4   **Prep Time:** 5 minutes   **Cook Time:** 10 minutes

When grilled, the lemon becomes extra sweet and juicy, and the Pistachio Mint Pesto is loaded with prebiotics. Serve with Wild Rice and Cranberry Pilaf (page 41) or a simple green salad.

4 bone-in lamb chops, about 6 to 8 ounces each

2 large garlic cloves, smashed

Sea salt

Freshly ground black pepper

1 tablespoon olive oil

2 lemons, halved

1 recipe Pistachio Mint Pesto (page 114)

1   Preheat a charcoal or gas grill or a grill pan to medium-high.

2   Rub the lamb with the garlic and then coat with olive oil, and season generously with salt and pepper.

3   Grill for 5 to 7 minutes on each side. Place the lemons cut-side down on the grill and cook until barely charred, about 10 minutes total, depending on the hotness of the grill. Serve the lamb with a generous spoonful of pesto and the grilled lemon halves.

9

SAUCES, DIPS, & SPREADS

Guacamole

Pico de Gallo

Mole

Arugula Pecan Pesto

Pistachio Mint Pesto

Chimichurri

Caper Gremolata

Chile de Arbol Salsa

Pomegranate Gremolata

Hummus

Roasted Red Pepper Hummus

Dukkah

Peanut Sauce

Sweet Chili Garlic Sauce

Barbecue Sauce

GUACAMOLE

Yields: 2 cups   **Prep Time:** 5 minutes   **Cook Time:** 0 minutes

Avocados are a rich source of polyols, fermentable carbohydrates. Whipped together with lime juice and garlic, they make a healthy, delicious addition to a wide variety of dishes or as a dip for vegetables.

6 ripe avocados, pitted

¼ teaspoon sea salt

2 tablespoons lime juice

2 garlic cloves, minced

½ jalapeño pepper, seeded and minced

1 plum tomato, seeded and diced

¼ cup minced fresh cilantro

1   Mash the avocado, sea salt, lime juice, garlic, and jalapeño in a mortar and pestle.

2   Stir in the tomato and cilantro. Serve immediately or press a round of parchment paper onto the surface and store in the refrigerator until ready to serve.

PICO DE GALLO

Yields: 4 cups   **Prep Time:** 10 minutes   **Cook Time:** 0 minutes

Once you learn to make your own salsa at home, you may never go back to store-bought. The best part about this salsa is that tomatoes have the best flavor when they're not refrigerated. Put it together within an hour of when you intend to serve it to let the flavors come together.

6 to 8 vine-ripened tomatoes, cored and diced

½ red onion, minced

2 garlic cloves, minced

1 jalapeño pepper, seeded and minced

2 tablespoons lime juice

¼ cup roughly chopped fresh cilantro

Sea salt

Freshly ground black pepper

Combine all of the ingredients in a non-reactive bowl. Season to taste with salt and pepper.

MOLE

Yields: 3 cups   **Prep Time:** 10 minutes   **Cook Time:** 45 minutes

Use this smoky, sweet sauce over Baja Bowls with Mole (page 90).

2 ounces dried pasilla chiles, stems and seeds removed

2 ounces dried guajillo chiles, stems and seeds removed

¼ cup sesame seeds

¼ cup blanched slivered almonds

1 tablespoon cumin seeds

1 tablespoon coriander seeds

2 tablespoons canola oil

2 yellow onions, thinly sliced

4 garlic cloves, minced

¼ cup raisins

1 teaspoon dried oregano

Zest and juice of 1 orange

2 cups Chicken Bone Broth (page 57) or vegetable broth

1 ounce bittersweet chocolate, grated

Sea salt

1   In a large, dry skillet over medium heat, toast the chiles until barely blackened, 2 to 3 minutes. Transfer them to a food processor or spice grinder.

2   Toast the sesame seeds for 1 to 2 minutes until golden brown. Transfer them to the food processor.

3   Toast the slivered almonds in a similar manner and transfer to the food processor.

4   Grind all of the ingredients to a fine powder in the food processor.

5   Toast the cumin and coriander seeds in the same skillet for 2 to 3 minutes, until fragrant. Transfer them to a mortar and pestle or spice grinder, and grind to a fine powder and add to the chile and sesame seed mixture.

6   In a large sauce pan, heat the canola oil over medium heat. Cook the onions with a pinch of salt until soft, about 15 minutes. Add the garlic and cook for another 2 minutes.

7   Add the raisins, oregano, orange juice and zest, and the ground spices and nuts. Pour in the broth. Bring to a simmer and cook for 30 minutes, until thick and fragrant. Stir in the chocolate until melted. Adjust seasoning to taste with salt.

ARUGULA PECAN PESTO

Yields: 1½ cups   **Prep Time:** 5 minutes   **Cook Time:** 0 minutes

Arugula, also known as rocket, has a peppery bite to it and is a great source of prebiotics. This pesto is perfect for topping grilled meats, dipping vegetables in, or slathering on crostini.

½ cup extra-virgin olive oil

3 garlic cloves, smashed

2 cups loosely packed fresh arugula

½ cup toasted pecans, roughly chopped

¼ teaspoon sea salt

¼ teaspoon freshly ground black pepper

Place all of the ingredients into a blender in the order listed. Pulse a few times, then stop the motor, and press down on the arugula with a spatula as needed to make sure the blades are reaching it. Blend until thoroughly integrated but still slightly chunky.

PISTACHIO MINT PESTO

Yields: 1 cup   **Prep Time:** 5 minutes   **Cook Time:** 0 minutes

Pistachios are a good source of resistant starch. This pesto is designed to accompany Grilled Lamb Chops with Pistachio Mint Pesto (page 109).

¼ cup extra-virgin olive oil

Juice of 1 lime

1 small shallot, minced

1 cup loosely packed fresh mint leaves

½ cup shelled roasted pistachios, roughly chopped

¼ teaspoon sea salt

¼ teaspoon freshly ground pepper

Place all of the ingredients into a blender in the order listed. Pulse a few times, then stop the motor and scrape down the sides. Blend until thoroughly integrated but still slightly chunky.

CHIMICHURRI

Yields: 1½ cups   **Prep Time:** 5 minutes   **Cook Time:** 0 minutes

Use this pungent sauce as both a marinade and a finishing sauce for grilled meat. Use raw apple cider vinegar for probiotic benefits.

¼ cup apple cider vinegar

½ teaspoon sea salt

Freshly ground black pepper

4 garlic cloves, minced

2 tablespoons minced red onion

¼ teaspoon red chile flakes

½ cup minced fresh flat-leaf parsley

2 tablespoons minced fresh oregano

¼ cup minced fresh cilantro

½ cup extra-virgin olive oil

Combine all of the ingredients except the olive oil in a glass bowl. Stir to combine. Slowly drizzle in the olive oil, whisking constantly to form an emulsion.

CAPER GREMOLATA

Serves: 2   **Prep Time:** 5 minutes   **Cook Time:** 0 minutes

This gremolata is delicious with grilled salmon. The brininess of the capers marries perfectly with the sweetness of the lemon and grassy parsley, and all are a great source of fermentable fibers.

¼ cup drained capers, minced

Zest and juice of 1 lemon

1 shallot, minced

½ cup minced fresh flat-leaf parsley

Pinch red chile flakes

Sea salt

1 Combine all of the ingredients in a non–reactive bowl.

2 Allow the flavors to marry for a few minutes before serving.

CHILE DE ARBOL SALSA

Yields: 4 cups   **Prep Time:** 5 minutes   **Cook Time:** 15 minutes

My neighbor Ludi taught me how to make this salsa. It's so fiery that she prepared the chiles on a portable stove on her back porch because of their intense aroma. Just open a window and you'll be fine. It's delicious with scrambled eggs, as a dip for corn tortilla chips, or, as Ludi advised, with basically anything you're eating. Chile peppers are filled with antioxidants, can boost immunity, and may improve mucous membranes, which can improve intestinal health.

2 cups husked tomatillos

2 cups plum tomatoes

2 jalapeño peppers

½ cup dried chile de arbol peppers, stems removed

Sea salt

1 Bring a large pot of salted water to a boil over medium heat. Cook the tomatillos, tomatoes, and jalapeño peppers until they're tender, about 10 minutes.

2 Allow to cool briefly. Remove the stems of the peppers. Place everything in a blender and purée until mostly smooth. Be careful to allow steam to escape occasionally without burning yourself.

3 Meanwhile, heat a large skillet over medium heat. Toast the chile de arbol peppers until browned but not blackened, shaking the skillet regularly. Grind them in a spice grinder and add to the blender. Blend until smooth.

4 Season to taste with salt.

POMEGRANATE GREMOLATA

Yields: 1½ cups   **Prep Time:** 10 minutes   **Cook Time:** 0 minutes

Prebiotics never tasted so delicious! This salsa, while not spicy in the traditional sense of the word, is perfect for topping roasted squash, pan-seared salmon, or lamb meatballs. If you've never broken apart a pomegranate before, don't worry—it's easy! Simply slice the fruit into quarters and turn the skin inside out. Peel back the papery white layers and gently brush your fingers across the arils (seeds), allowing them to fall into a bowl.

1 pomegranate, arils removed

1 cup roughly chopped fresh
flat-leaf parsley

1 large shallot, minced

¼ cup extra-virgin olive oil

Sea salt

Freshly ground black pepper

Combine all of the ingredients in a bowl, mixing to combine. Season with salt and pepper.

HUMMUS

Yields: 2 cups   **Prep Time:** 10 minutes, plus 8 hours inactive time
Cook Time: 1 to 2 hours

Although you can easily purchase prepared hummus in the grocery store, it costs exponentially more than homemade. Making it yourself also allows you to soak the chickpeas to improve their digestibility. Alternatively, rinse and drain a can of cooked chickpeas to use in this recipe.

1 cup dried chickpeas

¼ cup tahini

2 tablespoons extra-virgin olive oil

1 garlic clove

Juice of 1 lemon

Sea salt

Freshly ground black pepper

1 Soak the chickpeas overnight in several cups of fresh water. Rinse thoroughly.

2 Place the chickpeas in a sauce pan and cover with water. Bring to a simmer and cook for 1 to 2 hours, or until very tender.

3 Drain, reserving some of the cooking water.

4 Place the chickpeas in a blender along with the tahini, olive oil, garlic, and lemon juice. Purée until smooth, adding the reserved cooking water as needed to thin to the desired consistency. Season to taste with salt and pepper.

ROASTED RED PEPPER HUMMUS

Yields: 2 cups   **Prep Time:** 10 minutes, plus 8 hours inactive time
Cook Time: 1 to 2 hours

I love the beautiful smoky flavor of roasted red peppers and paprika in this tangy dip. Add more cayenne pepper for a bigger kick, if you like.

1 cup dried chickpeas

2 roasted red bell peppers, diced

2 tablespoons tahini

2 tablespoons extra-virgin olive oil

1 garlic clove

Juice of 1 lemon

1 teaspoon smoked paprika

¼ teaspoon cayenne pepper

Sea salt

Freshly ground black pepper

1 Soak the chickpeas overnight in several cups of fresh water. Rinse thoroughly.

2 Place the chickpeas in a sauce pan and cover with water. Bring to a simmer and cook for 1 to 2 hours, or until very tender.

3 Drain, reserving some of the cooking water.

4 Place the chickpeas in a blender along with the roasted red peppers, tahini, olive oil, garlic, lemon juice, paprika, and cayenne. Purée until smooth, adding the reserved cooking water as needed to thin to the desired consistency. Season to taste with salt and pepper.

DUKKAH

Yields: 1 cup   **Prep Time:** 5 minutes   **Cook Time:** 5 minutes

Dukkah, pronounced *doo-kah*, is a Middle Eastern combination of nuts, seeds, and spices. It's delicious as a coating for fish, a topping for roasted vegetables, or a dip for bread. Feel free to use alternative nuts or seeds, whatever you have on hand. I've used pistachios here because they're a good source of resistant starch.

1 tablespoon coriander seeds

1 tablespoon cumin seeds

½ teaspoon coarse sea salt

1 cup shelled pistachios

¼ cup sesame seeds

½ teaspoon dried mint

1 teaspoon dried parsley

1   Toast the coriander and cumin seeds in a dry skillet over medium heat until fragrant, about 2 minutes. Add them to a mortar and pestle or food processor. Add the salt and pistachios and bash until coarsely ground.

2   Toast the sesame seeds in the same skillet until gently browned, about 3 minutes. Remove from skillet and add them to the pistachio and spice mixture along with the mint and parsley. Stir to combine.

PEANUT SAUCE

Yields: 1 cup   **Prep Time:** 5 minutes   **Cook Time:** 5 minutes

Skip the bottled peanut sauces and opt for this healthier version. It's easy to whip up and delicious in stir-fries and for dipping spring rolls.

2 tablespoons toasted sesame oil

1 teaspoon minced ginger

1 teaspoon minced garlic

1 tablespoon sambal oelek chile sauce

¼ cup low-sodium, gluten-free soy sauce

2 tablespoons lime juice

¼ cup raw honey

½ cup natural peanut butter

1   Heat the sesame oil in a dry skillet over medium-low heat. Cook the ginger and garlic until fragrant, 1 to 2 minutes.

2   Add the sambal, soy sauce, lime juice, honey, and peanut butter to the skillet. Whisk until thoroughly integrated. Use immediately or place in a clean glass jar and store in the refrigerator for up to 3 days.

SWEET CHILI GARLIC SAUCE

Yields: 1 cup   **Prep Time:** 5 minutes   **Cook Time:** 5 minutes

Fresh chiles have antimicrobial properties and garlic is loaded with prebiotics. Sure, you could buy bottled chili sauce, but this version is simple to make and has less sugar than commercial varieties. Serve with Salad Rolls (page 33).

2 garlic cloves, minced

2 serrano peppers, cored and minced

¼ cup maple syrup

½ cup water, plus 1 tablespoon, divided

1 tablespoon cornstarch

¼ cup apple cider vinegar

1 Combine the garlic, serrano peppers, maple syrup, and water in a blender and purée until smooth.

2 Transfer the mixture to a small sauce pan and bring to a simmer over medium-low heat. In a small bowl, make a slurry with the cornstarch and the remaining tablespoon of water. Add the slurry to the sauce and cook until thickened, about 1 to 2 minutes. Remove the pan from the heat. Whisk in the apple cider vinegar.

3 Allow to cool completely before serving. Store in a covered container in the refrigerator for up to 3 days.

BARBECUE SAUCE

Yields: 2 cups   **Prep Time:** 5 minutes   **Cook Time:** 25 minutes

Although it's certainly easier to reach for a bottle of commercially prepared barbecue sauce, most are loaded with sugar or high-fructose corn syrup, neither of which is good for a healthy gut. Try this naturally sweetened low-sugar version instead.

1 yellow onion, minced

1 tablespoon olive oil

Pinch sea salt

2 garlic cloves, minced

1 (15-ounce) can tomato sauce

1 teaspoon Dijon mustard

2 fresh Medjool dates, pitted and diced

2 tablespoons apple cider vinegar

1 teaspoon smoked paprika

1 teaspoon ground cumin

¼ teaspoon cayenne pepper

Sea salt

Freshly ground black pepper

1 Cook the onion in a small sauce pan over medium-low heat along with the olive oil and a pinch of sea salt until soft and nearly caramelized, about 15 minutes. Add the garlic and cook for another 30 seconds.

2 Add all of the remaining ingredients and simmer uncovered for 10 minutes to allow all of the flavors to come together.

3 Adjust seasoning to taste with salt and pepper. For a smooth consistency, use an immersion blender to purée until smooth.

10

DESSERTS

Kombucha Granita

Berry Yogurt Popsicles

Frozen Banana Ice Cream with Cacao Nibs

Crustless Greek Yogurt Cheesecake

Cherry Compote

KOMBUCHA GRANITA

Serves: 2   **Prep Time:** 1½ minutes   **Cook Time:** 0 minutes

Kombucha is naturally sweet, with minimal sugar. It makes a delicious and healthy frozen dessert. Use homemade Basic Kombucha (page 77) or purchase some from the store in whatever flavor you like.

4 cups kombucha

Pour the kombucha into a shallow dish and place it in the freezer. Freeze for 30 minutes and then run the tines of a fork through the frozen edges, stirring them into the middle to create fine flakes. Return to the freezer and freeze for another 30 minutes. Repeat the process until the entire mixture is frozen, about 1½ hours. Serve with a spoon.

BERRY YOGURT POPSICLES

Serves: 4   **Prep Time:** 5 minutes   **Cook Time:** 0 minutes

Blueberries and raspberries are good sources of prebiotics and blend beautifully with yogurt. For a sweeter version, use the Honey Vanilla Yogurt (page 69) or opt for Greek Yogurt (page 70) for extra protein and creaminess.

2 cups blueberries   1 teaspoon vanilla extract
1 cup raspberries   4 cups yogurt

1 Combine the blueberries, raspberries, vanilla, and yogurt in a blender and purée until mostly smooth.

2 Pour the mixture into Popsicle molds and freeze until firm, about 2 hours. Submerge in warm water briefly to unmold.

FROZEN BANANA ICE CREAM WITH CACAO NIBS

Serves: 4   **Prep Time:** 5 minutes   **Cook Time:** 0 minutes

This recipe is so simple, but it satisfies my ice cream cravings without a hint of dairy or refined sugar. Both banana and cacao are good sources of prebiotics. It is best to prepare it immediately before you intend to serve, to prevent the bananas from browning.

3 cups frozen banana chunks

1½ cups unsweetened almond milk

1 teaspoon vanilla extract

Pinch sea salt

¼ cup cacao nibs or dark chocolate chips

1 Combine the banana chunks, almond milk, vanilla, and a pinch of sea salt in a blender. Purée until smooth, adding more almond milk as needed.

2 When it has reached the desired consistency, add the cacao nibs and pulse a few times just until integrated.

CRUSTLESS GREEK YOGURT CHEESECAKE

Serves: 4   **Prep Time:** 10 minutes, plus 4 to 6 hours inactive time
Cook Time: 0 minutes

This cheesecake does not require baking, which is a good thing because it keeps the probiotics in the yogurt intact. If possible, choose grass-fed gelatin, which is especially nourishing to your microbiome. Serve with Cherry Compote (page 129) and toasted crushed almonds.

2 teaspoons powdered gelatin

2 tablespoons warm water

2 cups Greek Yogurt (page 70)

8 ounces cream cheese, softened

½ cup raw honey

1 tablespoon vanilla extract

¼ teaspoon sea salt

1 Mix the gelatin and water in a small bowl to soften and set aside for 10 minutes.

2 Combine the yogurt, cream cheese, honey, vanilla, and sea salt in a blender and purée until thoroughly combined.

3 Stir the gelatin to make sure it is fully dissolved. Pour the softened gelatin into the blender and blend until thoroughly integrated.

4 Pour the mixture into a 6-inch springform pan. Tap to release any air bubbles. Cover tightly with plastic wrap and refrigerate for 4 to 6 hours, or until completely set.

CHERRY COMPOTE

Serves: 4   **Prep Time:** 5 minutes   **Cook Time:** 12 minutes

This resembles cherry pie filling but is so much better for you. The port is optional, but I love the complexity it brings to the sauce.

4 cups pitted cherries, fresh or frozen

¼ cup raw honey

¼ cup port (optional)

2 tablespoons tapioca flour

2 tablespoons water

1 Combine the cherries, honey, and port, if using, in a sauce pan over medium-low heat. If using frozen berries, watch the pan carefully to ensure they don't scorch.

2 Stir with a wooden spoon to break up the fruit. Cook for 10 minutes.

3 Dissolve the tapioca in the water and pour into the cherry mixture. Cook until just thickened, about 2 minutes. Allow to cool briefly before serving.

Part Three

GUT-HEALING RECIPES

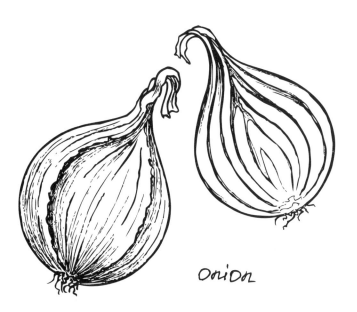

Onion

11

GUT-HEALING

The recipes here are in some ways opposite to the recipes in the previous section. They're still filled with healthy, whole foods, but they're designed to give your gut a rest. The recipes are free of grains, legumes, dairy, and refined sugar, and incorporate many of the underlying principles of the paleo, GAPS, Specific Carbohydrate, and Low-FODMAP diets. Cooking methods are designed to provide easily digestible, nourishing foods that pass through the small intestine and colon without feeding pathological bacteria or further damaging the lining of the gut. Whether you have small-intestinal bacterial overgrowth or recently diagnosed celiac disease, these dishes are easily digestible, help starve out the bad bacteria, and give your intestinal lining a chance to heal.

GUT CHECK

An imbalance in the gut microbiota may contribute to numerous gastrointestinal disorders, including irritable bowel syndrome, small intestinal bacterial overgrowth, leaky gut, and inflammatory bowel diseases.

IRRITABLE BOWEL SYNDROME

Whether or not you have been diagnosed with irritable bowel syndrome (IBS), chances are you have experienced symptoms of the disease at some point in your life: abdominal pain, cramping, bloating, gas, diarrhea, and constipation. Symptoms can occur as a result of chronic or acute stress, poor nutrition, infection, or changes in the microbiota.

SMALL INTESTINAL BACTERIAL OVERGROWTH

Small intestinal bacterial overgrowth (SIBO) is a possible cause for irritable bowel syndrome. As its name suggests, SIBO involves an overgrowth of bacteria in the small intestine and may also involve the relocation of bacteria that belong in the colon into the small intestine. A low-FODMAP diet is one treatment option for SIBO and involves temporarily eliminating many of the foods described in the preceding section of this book (those with fermentable fibers) until the microbiota returns to a state of balance. It may also involve a course of antibiotics specifically designed to stay within the gastrointestinal tract.

LEAKY GUT

The gastrointestinal tract is the primary barrier between our internal and the external worlds and protects the body from external substances—including those we ingest. A "leaky" gut fails to do this. According to the book *Bugs, Bowels, and Behavior,* "The intestinal mucosal barrier heavily influences the immune response that begins with and results from antigen interaction. If this complex intestinal barrier is broken, foreign molecules can enter, interact with the immune system, and launch an inflammatory response that can lead to a multitude of local intestinal as well as systemic extra-intestinal diseases."

Symptoms of leaky gut include diarrhea, constipation, gas, bloating, nutritional deficiencies, compromised immunity, headaches, brain fog, and chronic fatigue.

INFLAMMATORY BOWEL DISEASE

The two most common types of inflammatory bowel disease (IBD) are Crohn's and ulcerative colitis, which are autoimmune diseases. Symptoms are often severe and debilitating and include diarrhea, abdominal pain, bleeding, weight loss, and anemia. It is very important to seek the advice of a primary care physician and gastroenterologist if you suspect that you have an inflammatory bowel disease.

NUTRITION FOR HEALING

Conventional therapies for both IBS and IBD may involve dietary modifications, stress reduction, and antibiotics. Severe cases of IBD may require more serious interventions including surgery to remove the damaged section of the intestine.

The Specific Carbohydrate Diet is a novel nutritional approach to treating gastrointestinal disorders developed by Dr. Sidney V. Haas in 1924 and later built upon by Elaine Gottschall in the book *Breaking the Vicious Cycle*. The diet allows easily digestible monosaccharides along with healthy sources of fat and protein. It eliminates grains, starchy vegetables, lactose-containing dairy products, and legumes.

The GAPS diet is similar to Specific Carbohydrate but incorporates more probiotic foods, as well as other unique features.

The low-FODMAP diet eliminates or drastically reduces foods containing fermentable carbohydrates (yes, all of the foods included in abundance in Part Two of this book). A low-FODMAP diet improves symptoms of IBD for many individuals. However, eventually foods containing FODMAPs should be reintroduced in small amounts as tolerance increases.

The ultimate goal of these diets is to return the microbiota to a state of health and balance, prevent further damage to the gastrointestinal tract, and bring healing to damaged intestinal lumen.

Note: I am a cook, not a doctor. If you have or suspect you have irritable bowel disease or any other medical condition, seek the advice of your primary care physician. This book is in no way intended to diagnose, treat, prevent, or cure any disease, nor is it intended to replace the advice of a medical doctor.

12

GUT-HEALING BREAKFASTS

MEDITERRANEAN VEGETABLE SCRAMBLE

Serves: 2   **Prep Time:** 5 minutes   **Cook Time:** 5 minutes

This scramble combines low-FODMAP vegetables with protein and fat from eggs for a filling and delicious breakfast. The fresh herbs are optional, but they do improve the flavor and are easily digestible.

1 teaspoon extra-virgin olive oil

1 cup diced zucchini

½ cup diced tomatoes

1 tablespoon minced fresh basil

4 eggs, whisked

Sea salt

Freshly ground black pepper

1 Heat the olive oil in a small skillet over medium heat. Sauté the zucchini for 2 minutes, until golden but not browned.

2 Add the tomatoes and basil and cook for 30 seconds.

3 Reduce the heat to low. Pour in the eggs, season generously with salt and pepper, and cook until the eggs are set, stirring constantly with a spatula.

HAM AND SPINACH SCRAMBLE

Serves: 1   **Prep Time:** 5 minutes   **Cook Time:** 5 minutes

This scramble has a bit more protein than the Mediterranean veggie scramble. For vegetarians, omit the ham and replace with ¼ cup diced red bell pepper.

1 teaspoon extra-virgin olive oil

¼ cup diced uncured cooked ham

1 cup roughly chopped fresh spinach

1 green onion (green parts only) thinly sliced

2 eggs, whisked

Sea salt

Freshly ground black pepper

1 Heat the olive oil in a small skillet over medium heat.

2 Cook the diced ham, spinach, and green onion until the spinach is soft and most of the moisture has evaporated, about 5 minutes.

3 Reduce the heat to low. Pour in the eggs, season generously with salt and pepper, and cook until the eggs are set, stirring constantly with a spatula.

BACON, ROASTED RED PEPPER, AND SPINACH FRITTATA

Serves: 2 to 4   **Prep Time:** 5 minutes   **Cook Time:** 25 to 30 minutes

Make sure to choose uncured bacon without added sugar or artificial chemicals. Onions and garlic contain FODMAPs, so read labels carefully if you find that they are difficult for you to digest. The green portion of green onions is a delicious low-FODMAP alternative. For vegetarians, replace the bacon fat with 1 tablespoon of olive oil.

2 slices uncured bacon, cut into thin strips

2 roasted red bell peppers, drained and cut into thin strips

2 tablespoons green onions (green parts only) thinly sliced

1 teaspoon fresh thyme leaves

2 cups fresh spinach, roughly chopped

6 eggs, whisked

Sea salt

Freshly ground black pepper

1 Preheat the oven to 375°F.

2 Heat a medium ovenproof skillet over medium–low heat and cook the bacon for 5 to 10 minutes, until it has rendered most of its fat.

3 Add the peppers, green onions, thyme, and spinach. Cook until the spinach is soft and most of the liquid has evaporated, about 5 minutes.

4 Add the eggs, season with salt and pepper, and cook undisturbed for another 2 to 3 minutes, just until the edges are set.

5 Place the entire pan into the oven and bake for 10 to 15 minutes, or until the eggs are cooked through. Slice and serve.

FARMER'S MARKET VEGETABLE HASH

Serves: 2   **Prep Time:** 5 minutes   **Cook Time:** 40 minutes

I find that when I make this filling, delicious breakfast hash, I'm not hungry for hours afterward. As your gut heals, you may find that you can handle the sweet potato unpeeled, or swap in some white potatoes. I like to serve this with a couple of poached eggs.

1 large sweet potato, peeled and cut into ½-inch dice

1 small zucchini, cut into 1-inch dice

1 red bell pepper, cored and thinly sliced

¼ fennel bulb, thinly sliced

1 rosemary sprig, needles only, minced

1 to 2 tablespoons coconut oil

Sea salt

Freshly ground black pepper

1 Preheat the oven to 375°F.

2 Spread the sweet potato, zucchini, bell pepper, fennel, and rosemary on a sheet pan. Coat with the coconut oil and season with salt and pepper. Roast uncovered for 30 minutes.

3 Flip the vegetables with a metal spatula. Return to the oven to cook for another 10 minutes.

APPLE SAUSAGE AND BUTTERNUT SQUASH HASH

Serves: 4   **Prep Time:** 10 minutes   **Cook Time:** 30 to 40 minutes

Save time in your morning routine by prepping all of these ingredients the night before. If you prefer not to peel and dice a whole butternut squash, check the chilled case of the produce section for precut butternut squash. For low-FODMAP, choose a sausage without apple. Replace the apple and onion in the recipe with an additional cup of butternut squash.

4 chicken apple sausages, sliced into 1-inch pieces

2 cups cubed butternut squash

2 Golden Delicious apples, peeled and cut into 1-inch pieces

1 yellow onion, halved and thinly sliced

3 tablespoons extra-virgin olive oil, divided

Sea salt

Freshly ground black pepper

2 cups roughly chopped fresh spinach

4 eggs

1   Preheat the oven to 375°F.

2   Spread the apple sausages, butternut squash, apples, and onion on a rimmed baking sheet. Drizzle with 2 tablespoons of the olive oil. Toss to coat and then season with salt and pepper. Roast uncovered for 30 to 40 minutes, or until the squash is tender and gently browned.

3   Remove the pan from the oven and toss with the spinach, just to wilt it.

4   During the last 5 minutes of cooking, heat the remaining olive oil in a large skillet over medium–high heat. Fry the eggs until the whites are set and the yolks are still runny.

5   Divide the hash between individual bowls and top each portion with a fried egg.

SPAGHETTI SQUASH HASH BROWNS

Serves: 2   **Prep Time:** 5 minutes   **Cook Time:** 50 minutes

If you're craving hash browns but cannot enjoy white potatoes, look no further than spaghetti squash. Prepare the spaghetti squash the night before with whatever you're making for dinner to make breakfast prep a breeze.

1 spaghetti squash

Sea salt

Freshly ground black pepper

2 tablespoons extra-virgin olive oil

1 Preheat the oven to 350°F.

2 Slice the spaghetti squash in half lengthwise and scoop out the seeds. Place it cut-side down in a baking dish. Roast uncovered for 40 minutes. Scoop out the flesh with a fork. Allow to cool completely.

3 Form the spaghetti squash into 4 to 6 small patties. Squeeze out any excess moisture, as you would with fresh hash browns. Season with salt and pepper.

4 Heat the oil in a large skillet. Pan-fry on each side for about 4 minutes or until gently browned.

BLUEBERRY BANANA PANCAKES

Serves: 4   **Prep Time:** 5 minutes   **Cook Time:** 15 minutes

This is one of my family's favorite breakfasts. It's also delicious with a scoop of coconut cream or a small drizzle of maple syrup.

6 eggs

1¼ cups almond meal

2 ripe bananas

1 teaspoon baking soda

⅛ teaspoon sea salt

Zest of 1 lemon

¼ teaspoon freshly grated nutmeg

1 cup blueberries

2 tablespoons coconut oil or palm shortening

1 Combine all of the ingredients except the blueberries and oil in a blender. Pulse until smooth, scraping down the sides with a spatula to ensure the batter is thoroughly combined. Add the blueberries and pulse once or twice, until just incorporated.

2 Heat a large skillet over medium-low heat. Melt the coconut oil and tilt the pan to coat.

3 Pour the batter into the pan in 3 small circles, 2 to 3 tablespoons per pancake. Cook until bubbles begin to appear in the center of each, about 3 minutes. Flip carefully. The pancake will still be very loose. Cook on the other side for 1 minute. Serve immediately or transfer to a dish in a warm oven until all are cooked. Repeat with the remaining batter.

GRAIN-FREE CREPES

Yields: 8 to 10 crepes **Prep Time:** 5 minutes **Cook Time:** 10 minutes

Take these crepes in a sweet or savory direction. Or, use them as wraps for enchiladas.

1 cup coconut milk

3 eggs

1 teaspoon vanilla extract, for sweet crepes

½ cup arrowroot powder

2 teaspoons baking powder

Generous pinch sea salt

2 tablespoons coconut oil

1 Combine the coconut milk, eggs, and vanilla, if using, in a blender. Blend until smooth.

2 Add the arrowroot, baking powder, and a generous pinch of sea salt. Pulse a few times, scrape down the sides, and then blend until integrated.

3 Heat a small skillet over medium heat until hot. Add 1 to 2 teaspoons coconut oil and swirl to coat the pan.

4 Pour about ¼ cup of the crepe batter into the pan, tilting to coat the bottom of the pan. Cook until the top is set, about 2 minutes, and then flip gently to cook on the other side for 1 minute. Slide the crepe onto a parchment paper–lined dish.

5 Repeat the process with the remaining crepes.

SAVORY ASPARAGUS CREPES WITH HOLLANDAISE

Serves: 4   **Prep Time:** 5 minutes   **Cook Time:** 10 minutes

Ghee is more easily digestible for people with dairy intolerance because it contains virtually no lactose or casein but pure butterfat. However, if you're sensitive to it, use another neutral oil such as macadamia or avocado oil.

1 bunch asparagus, woody ends trimmed

3 egg yolks

Pinch sea salt

2 teaspoons lemon juice

⅓ cup melted ghee

1 recipe Grain-Free Crepes (page 145)

1 Heat a large pot of salted water over high heat. Plunge the asparagus into the water for about 3 minutes, until bright green and barely tender. Drain thoroughly.

2 Place the egg yolks, salt, and lemon juice in a small sauce pot over low heat. Whisk until pale yellow. Slowly drizzle in the ghee, whisking constantly until all of it is incorporated.

3 Divide the asparagus between the crepes and fold them as desired. Drizzle with the hollandaise sauce and serve immediately.

CARAMELIZED BANANA CINNAMON STUFFED CREPES

Serves: 4   **Prep Time:** 5 minutes   **Cook Time:** 10 minutes

These decadent crepes will satisfy your cravings for something sweet. Cooking the bananas makes them more easily digestible and intensifies their sweetness.

2 tablespoons ghee or coconut oil

3 just-ripe bananas, sliced in ½-inch-thick rounds

¼ cup orange juice

¼ teaspoon ground cinnamon

¼ teaspoon freshly ground nutmeg

Sea salt

1 recipe Grain-Free Crepes (page 145)

1 Heat the ghee in a large skillet over medium heat. Place the bananas cut-side down in the skillet and brown on each side for about 3 minutes.

2 Add the orange juice, cinnamon, nutmeg, and a small pinch of salt. Swirl this around the pan and ladle it over the bananas. Cook until the sauce thickens slightly, about 2 to 3 minutes.

3 Fill the crepes with the banana mixture and fold as desired.

ALMOND GRANOLA

Yields: 5 cups   **Prep Time:** 10 minutes, plus 8 hours inactive time
Cook Time: 30 minutes, plus 1 hour resting time

Sometimes on a grain- and dairy-free diet, you just crave a nice cold cereal. This granola contains no oats at all, making it gentler on your digestive system. Definitely soak the nuts ahead of time to improve digestibility.

2 cups almonds

1 cup walnuts

1 cup cashews

½ teaspoon sea salt, divided

1 tablespoon vanilla extract

1 teaspoon ground cinnamon

¼ to ½ cup maple syrup

1 cup unsweetened shredded coconut

1 Combine the almonds, walnuts, and cashews in a large container and cover with fresh water and ¼ teaspoon of the salt. Allow to soak overnight at room temperature.

2 Rinse and drain the nuts thoroughly, until the water runs clear. Spread them out on a mesh rack or pan lined with paper towels and allow them to air dry.

3 Preheat the oven to 350°F.

4 Combine the nuts, the remaining ¼ teaspoon of salt, and the vanilla, cinnamon, and maple syrup in a food processor, adding more maple syrup until it reaches your desired level of sweetness. Pulse until coarsely ground. Add the shredded coconut and pulse until just combined.

5 Spread the mixture out onto a rimmed baking tray. Bake for 15 minutes. Stir with a metal spatula. Bake for another 15 minutes. Stir again. Turn off the oven and allow the granola to stay in the oven for another hour to continue drying out.

6 Allow to cool completely before storing in an airtight container in the refrigerator. Serve with almond milk and fresh berries.

MACADAMIA CRANBERRY GRANOLA

Yields: 5 cups   **Prep Time:** 5 minutes   **Cook Time:** 35 minutes

This granola is the epitome of decadence. The macadamia nuts are packed with gut-nourishing fats offset by the sweet, tart cranberries.

2 cups toasted macadamia nuts

¼ teaspoon sea salt

1 teaspoon vanilla extract

¼ cup maple syrup

2 cups unsweetened shredded coconut

1 cup unsweetened dried cranberries

1 Preheat the oven to 350°F.

2 Combine the macadamia nuts, salt, vanilla, and maple syrup in a food processor. Pulse until coarsely ground. Add the shredded coconut and pulse until just combined.

3 Spread the mixture onto a rimmed baking tray and press down as if forming a granola bar. Bake for 20 minutes. Break apart the bar with a metal spatula, flipping the pieces over. Bake for another 15 minutes.

4 Remove the pan from the oven and stir in the dried cranberries.

5 Allow to cool completely before storing in an airtight container in the refrigerator. Serve with almond milk.

BANANA PECAN MUFFINS

Yields: 12   **Prep Time:** 10 minutes   **Cook Time:** 15 to 18 minutes

Cooked fruit is often easier to digest than raw because the sugars are broken down and more easily absorbed. Bananas are a low-FODMAP fruit that do triple duty in this simple muffin recipe—they sweeten, provide structure, and improve texture.

1 cup cashew butter

2 eggs

2 overripe bananas

1½ teaspoons apple cider vinegar

2 teaspoons vanilla extract

1 teaspoon ground cinnamon

½ teaspoon ground nutmeg

¼ teaspoon sea salt

1 teaspoon baking soda

1 cup toasted pecan pieces

1 Preheat the oven to 350°F. Line a 12-cup muffin tin with paper liners.

2 Combine the cashew butter, eggs, bananas, apple cider vinegar, and vanilla in a food processor. Blend until smooth.

3 Add the cinnamon, nutmeg, salt, and baking soda and blend until smooth. Fold in the pecan pieces. Immediately pour the mixture into the prepared muffin tin.

4 Bake for 15 to 18 minutes, until the tops are golden brown and a toothpick inserted in the center comes out clean.

13

GUT-HEALING ENTRÉES

Basic Roasted Chicken

Herb and Lemon Roasted Chicken

Spanish Chicken Stew

Coq au Vin

Chicken with Stewed Vegetables

Duck Leg with Boysenberry Glaze

Duck Breast and Ginger Honey Endive

Pork Chops with Olive Tapenade

Pork Sirloin with Roasted Tomatoes

Ratatouille with Seared Ahi Tuna

Poached Halibut and French Vegetables

Shrimp Scampi

Salmon with Honey Dijon Baby Bok Choy

Steamed Mussels

Shrimp and Collards

Prosciutto-Wrapped Scallops

Beef Bourguignon

Burger Stacks with Caramelized Onions

Beef and Green Bean Stir-Fry

Steak and Vegetable Shish Kebabs

BASIC ROASTED CHICKEN

Serves: 4   **Prep Time:** 5 minutes   **Cook Time:** 45 to 60 minutes

Roasting a whole chicken is a little intimidating at first, especially prepared "spatchcock," but it's deceptively easy and the bird cooks quickly and evenly. As a bonus, once you learn how to do it, you'll have everything you need for a quick chicken stock and enjoy good-quality chicken for a fraction of the cost of meat that has already been cut into pieces.

1 (3- to 4-pound) whole chicken, preferably organic and free-range

2 tablespoons extra-virgin olive oil

Sea salt

Freshly ground black pepper

1 Preheat the oven to 375°F.

2 Place the chicken breast-side down on a cutting board, then lift the open end toward you. Using a sharp pair of kitchen shears, cut down each side of the backbone. Be careful to keep your fingers away from the cutting blade. Alternatively, use a sharp serrated knife and angle the open end of the chicken away from you. Reserve the backbone for making stock.

3 Place the chicken breast-side up on a roasting pan, opening it up so that the inside of the chicken is touching the pan. Flatten the bird with the palm of your hand.

4 Coat it generously with oil and then season on all sides with salt and pepper.

5 Roast uncovered for 45 minutes to 1 hour, or until the chicken is cooked through to an internal temperature of 160°F. It will continue cooking after you pull it out of the oven. Allow it to rest for at least 10 minutes before carving.

HERB AND LEMON ROASTED CHICKEN

Serves: 2 to 4   **Prep Time:** 5 minutes   **Cook Time:** 1 to 1½ hours

The flavors of lemon zest and herbs permeate the chicken and vegetables in this one-pan chicken recipe. With the tender stewed vegetables, it makes a delicious complete meal.

½ cup roughly chopped fresh flat-leaf parsley

¼ cup fresh thyme leaves

2 tablespoons fresh rosemary needles

1 lemon

6 tablespoons extra-virgin olive oil, divided

1 (3- to 4-pound) whole chicken, preferably organic and free-range

4 plum tomatoes, halved

1 red onion, sliced in thick rings

2 medium zucchini, sliced in 1-inch rounds

10 garlic cloves, smashed

Sea salt

Freshly ground black pepper

1 Preheat the oven to 375°F.

2 Combine the parsley, thyme, and rosemary in a blender. Zest the lemon and add the zest to the blender along with 4 tablespoons of the olive oil. Pulse the mixture until it forms a thick paste.

3 Place the chicken breast-side up on a roasting pan. Season the interior cavity with salt and pepper. Cut the lemon in half and stuff the halves inside the bird.

4 Season the exterior of the chicken liberally with salt and pepper, then coat it with the herb paste.

5 Scatter the tomatoes, onion, zucchini, and garlic around the chicken. Drizzle with the remaining 2 tablespoons of olive oil and season with salt and pepper.

6 Roast uncovered for 1 to 1½ hours, or until the chicken is cooked through to an internal temperature of 160°F. It will continue cooking after you pull it out of the oven. Allow it to rest for at least 10 minutes before carving.

SPANISH CHICKEN STEW

Serves: 4 to 6   **Prep Time:** 5 minutes
Cook Time: 25 to 30 minutes

The soft-cooked vegetables in this dish are flavorful and comforting. For a low-FODMAP version, omit the garlic and onion.

2 tablespoons extra-virgin olive oil

8 skinless, bone-in chicken thighs

1 yellow onion, halved and thinly sliced

1 red bell pepper, cored and thinly sliced

1 green bell pepper, cored and thinly sliced

2 garlic cloves, smashed

½ cup pepper-stuffed olives

1 teaspoon smoked paprika

½ teaspoon ground coriander

1 tablespoon tomato paste

2 quarts (8 cups) Chicken Bone Broth (page 57)

1 tablespoon red wine vinegar

¼ cup roughly chopped fresh flat-leaf parsley, for serving

2 lemons, cut into wedges, for serving

Sea salt

Freshly ground black pepper

1   Heat the olive oil in a large pot over medium–high heat. Season the chicken thighs with salt and pepper. Cook for 1 to 2 minutes on each side to brown. Remove the chicken to a plate to rest. It will not be cooked through at this point.

2   In the same pot, sauté the onion and peppers for 3 minutes. Add the garlic, olives, paprika, coriander, tomato paste, broth, and vinegar. Bring to a simmer and return the chicken thighs to the pot. Cover and cook on medium–low until the chicken is cooked through, about 20 minutes. Season with salt and pepper to taste.

3   Serve with fresh parsley and lemon wedges.

COQ AU VIN

Serves: 4 **Prep Time:** 5 minutes **Cook Time:** 1 hour

Chicken stewed in wine is a classic French technique that tenderizes the meat. I prefer to use white wine because I think the chicken looks prettier that way and I like the wine's delicate flavor. Virtually all of the alcohol cooks out.

2 tablespoons extra-virgin olive oil

4 skinless, bone-in chicken breasts, about 8 to 12 ounces each

2 garlic cloves, smashed

4 shallots, peeled and quartered lengthwise

4 thyme sprigs

1 cup Chicken Bone Broth (page 57)

2 cups dry white wine

Sea salt

Freshly ground black pepper

1 Heat the olive oil in a large, wide-bottomed pot. Season the chicken on all sides with salt and pepper. Place top-side down and sear until well browned, about 5 minutes. Flip the chicken and brown on the other side for 5 minutes.

2 Add the garlic and shallots to the pan and cook for 2 minutes.

3 Add the thyme sprigs and then pour in the chicken broth and white wine. Bring to a simmer. Cover and cook on medium-low heat for 45 to 50 minutes, or until the chicken is very tender and cooked through.

CHICKEN
WITH STEWED VEGETABLES

Serves: 2 to 4   **Prep Time:** 5 minutes   **Cook Time:** 45 minutes

These vegetables have a soft, creamy consistency that's both delicious and easy to digest.

2 tablespoons extra-virgin olive oil

4 to 6 skinless, bone-in chicken thighs, about 8 to 12 ounces each

Sea salt

Freshly ground black pepper

1 yellow onion, halved and thinly sliced

1 medium zucchini, quartered lengthwise and cut into ½-inch pieces

1 pint grape tomatoes

2 garlic cloves, smashed

2 thyme sprigs

1 rosemary sprig

½ cup dry red wine

1 Heat the olive oil in a large, wide-bottomed pot. Season the chicken on all sides with salt and pepper. Place top-side down and sear until well browned, about 5 minutes. Flip the chicken and brown on the other side for 5 minutes.

2 Add the onion, zucchini, tomatoes, garlic, thyme, and rosemary to the pan and cook for 2 minutes.

3 Pour in the red wine. Bring to a simmer. Cover and cook on medium-low heat for 35 minutes, or until the chicken is very tender and cooked through.

DUCK LEG WITH BOYSENBERRY GLAZE

Serves: 2   **Prep Time:** 10 minutes   **Cook Time:** 35 to 40 minutes

I enjoyed this dish originally at a small pub in rural England, where my son's preschool hosted a regular mum's night out. What a brilliant idea! Boysenberries are a low-FODMAP fruit, but you could also use whatever fruit happens to be in season.

2 tablespoons duck fat or olive oil

2 bone-in, skin-on duck legs, about 8 ounces each

Sea salt

Freshly ground pepper

1 cup boysenberries or blackberries

1 rosemary sprig

1 tablespoon tapioca starch

1 tablespoon water

1 Preheat the oven to 350°F.

2 Heat a large ovenproof skillet over medium-high heat and melt the duck fat.

3 Thoroughly dry the duck legs and then season with salt and pepper. Sear the duck skin-side down for 4 to 5 minutes, until browned.

4 Flip the duck and cook for another 2 minutes.

5 Place the pan in the oven and roast for another 25 to 30 minutes, or until the duck is cooked through to an internal temperature of 170°F.

6 Meanwhile, place the boysenberries and rosemary in a small sauce pan over medium-low heat.

7 Mash with a potato masher to release the juices from the fruit. Allow to cook for 10 minutes. Strain the mixture and return it to the pan.

8 In a small bowl, make a slurry with the tapioca starch and water. Pour it into the boysenberry sauce and whisk, cooking until just thickened. Remove from the heat.

9 Remove the duck from the oven and allow to rest for at least 5 minutes before serving. Drizzle the blackberry sauce over each plate and top with the duck legs.

DUCK BREAST AND GINGER HONEY ENDIVE

Serves: 4 **Prep Time:** 5 minutes **Cook Time:** 1 hour, 5 to 10 minutes

Endive is a good source of prebiotics and its bitterness is mellowed by a long, slow roast and a drizzle of honey.

6 heads Belgian endive

¼ cup extra-virgin olive oil

Sea salt

Freshly ground black pepper

4 skin-on duck breasts, about 6 to 8 ounces each

1 tablespoon minced ginger

1 teaspoon minced garlic

1 tablespoon honey

1 Preheat the oven to 425°F.

2 Trim the ends from each endive bulb and discard any discolored outer leaves. Slice in half lengthwise. Place the endive on a rimmed baking sheet and drizzle with the olive oil. Toss to coat thoroughly. Season with salt and pepper. Roast uncovered for 50 to 60 minutes.

3 Meanwhile, score the duck breasts by cutting through the skin in a diamond pattern at 1-inch intervals. Do not cut all the way through to the meat.

4 During the last 20 minutes of the endive's roasting time, heat a large skillet over medium-high heat. Sear the duck breast, skin-side down, until it renders some of its fat, about 5 to 7 minutes.

5 Remove the endive from the oven and toss with the ginger, garlic, and honey. Make space on the pan for the duck breasts and place them skin-side up on the pan. Roast for another 10 minutes, or until the duck is cooked to your desired level of doneness. Allow to rest for 5 minutes before slicing and serving.

PORK CHOPS WITH OLIVE TAPENADE

Serves: 2   **Prep Time:** 10 minutes, plus 30 minutes to 4 hours inactive time   **Cook Time:** 15 to 20 minutes

A quick brine will make your pork chops deliciously moist and juicy. They're delicious topped with a briny olive tapenade and over a bed of mixed greens.

1 tablespoon peppercorns

1 garlic clove, mashed

2 tablespoons sea salt, plus more for seasoning

2 tablespoons red wine vinegar

2 cups water

4 bone-in pork chops, about 6 to 8 ounces each

1 cup pitted mixed olives

2 tablespoons extra-virgin olive oil, plus more for step 4

2 tablespoons minced fresh flat-leaf parsley

2 tablespoons minced capers

Zest and juice of one lemon

4 cups mixed baby greens, for serving

Freshly ground black pepper

1 Combine the peppercorns, garlic, salt, vinegar, and water in a non-reactive dish. Stir to dissolve the salt. Place the pork chops into the brine and allow to rest for at least 30 minutes or up to 4 hours in the refrigerator.

2 Preheat the oven to 400°F.

3 Remove the pork from the brine and pat dry with paper towels.

4 Rub with olive oil and season with salt and pepper.

5 Heat a large, ovenproof skillet over medium-high heat until very hot.

6 Sear the pork chops on one side until browned, about 3 to 4 minutes. Flip the pork and transfer the skillet to the oven for 7 to 10 minutes, or until the pork is cooked through to an internal temperature of 140 to 145°F. Allow to rest for 5 minutes before serving.

7 While the pork chops are finishing in the oven, combine the olives, olive oil, parsley, capers, and lemon in a food processor. Pulse a few times, until chunky and thoroughly integrated. To serve, divide the mixed greens between serving dishes. Top with a pork chop and a dollop of the olive tapenade.

PORK SIRLOIN
WITH ROASTED TOMATOES

Serves: 4   **Prep Time:** 10 minutes   **Cook Time:** 60 minutes

Roasting brings out the inherent sweetness in tomatoes and increases the bioavailability of lycopene. This dish is delicious served with Mashed Parsnips (page 176). For low-FODMAP, omit the garlic.

1 boneless pork sirloin roast, about 2 pounds

4 tablespoons extra-virgin olive oil, divided

2 pounds ripe tomatoes

4 thyme sprigs

1 rosemary sprig, needles removed

4 garlic cloves, smashed

Sea salt

Freshly ground black pepper

1 Preheat the oven to 375°F.

2 Coat the pork sirloin with 2 tablespoons of olive oil. Season on all sides with salt and pepper. Place it in the center of a large, rimmed baking sheet.

3 Cut the tomatoes in half. In a large bowl, toss them with the remaining 2 tablespoons of olive oil, the thyme and rosemary, and the garlic. Season generously with salt and pepper.

4 Spread the tomatoes on the sheet pan, cut-side up.

5 Roast uncovered for 60 minutes, until the pork is cooked through to an internal temperature of 140 to 145°F and the tomatoes are caramelized.

RATATOUILLE WITH SEARED AHI TUNA

Serves: 4   **Prep Time:** 10 minutes   **Cook Time:** 1 hour to 1 hour 10 minutes

Seared ahi tuna and ratatouille are perhaps an unlikely pair, but the flavors are exquisite together. They make a delicious Mediterranean paleo, low-carb dinner that's brimming with gut-nourishing omega-3s and loads of brightly colored vegetables. The anchovy paste is optional, but it does add a briny depth of flavor to the ratatouille. For low-FODMAP, omit the garlic and onion.

½ cup extra-virgin olive oil, divided

1 eggplant, cut into 1-inch cubes

2 medium zucchini, cut into 1-inch rounds

1 yellow onion, diced

4 garlic cloves, minced

1 teaspoon anchovy paste (optional)

4 vine-ripened tomatoes

1 tablespoon fresh thyme leaves

½ cup roughly chopped fresh flat-leaf parsley

2 tablespoons balsamic vinegar

4 ahi tuna steaks, about 8 ounces each

Sea salt

Freshly ground black pepper

1   Preheat the oven to 325°F.

2   In a large skillet, heat ¼ cup of the olive oil over medium heat. When it is hot, add the eggplant and season generously with salt and pepper. Cook for about 10 minutes, until browned. Transfer the eggplant to a 2–quart baking dish.

3   Add another 2 tablespoons of olive oil to the pan and cook the zucchini until browned, about 5 to 10 minutes. Transfer it to the baking dish with the eggplant.

4   Cook the onion, garlic, and anchovy paste, if using, in the same pan for 10 to 15 minutes, until the onion is beginning to brown and caramelize. Add the tomatoes, thyme, and parsley and cook for another 5 minutes. Transfer the mixture to the baking dish, add the balsamic vinegar, and give everything a good toss. These steps can be done ahead of time if you like and stored in the refrigerator until ready to serve.

5 Place the ratatouille in the oven and bake for another 20 minutes, or 40 minutes if it was refrigerated. Allow to rest for 10 minutes before serving.

6 After the ratatouille is out of the oven, cook the fish. In a clean skillet, heat the remaining 2 tablespoons of olive oil over medium-high heat. Pat the tuna steaks dry with paper towels and season generously with salt and pepper. When the pan is hot, sear on each side for 2 to 3 minutes. The thicker the steak, the longer it will take. However, be sure not to overcook the fish. It should still be dark pink on the inside.

POACHED HALIBUT
AND FRENCH VEGETABLES

Serves: 4   **Prep Time:** 10 minutes   **Cook Time:** 30 to 35 minutes

Spring vegetables and tender halibut make an elegant French meal. This recipe is adapted from a dish shared in *Saveur* magazine, but I've streamlined the preparation and added fish for a filling and healthy entrée. Blanching and shocking the vegetables retains both their bright color and their nutritional value.

2 carrots, peeled, halved lengthwise and cut into 2-inch pieces

1 bunch asparagus, woody ends trimmed

¼ cup extra-virgin olive oil, divided

1 fennel bulb, cut into eighths

2 shallots, peeled and halved vertically

5 garlic cloves, smashed

½ cup vegetable broth

1 tablespoon sherry vinegar

1 vanilla bean pod, split lengthwise

4 halibut fillets, about 5 ounces each

Sea salt

Freshly ground black pepper

2 cups snow peas, strings removed

1 Bring a large pot of salted water to a boil. Prepare an ice-water bath in a large bowl. Blanch the carrots in the boiling water for 3 to 4 minutes, until slightly softened. Plunge into the ice water to stop the cooking process, and then drain.

2 Return the water to a boil and repeat the process with the asparagus, cooking for 1 to 2 minutes, until bright green. Plunge into the ice-water bath and then drain. These steps can be done ahead of time.

3 Warm the olive oil in a large skillet over medium heat. Brown the fennel for about 5 minutes on each side. Remove it to a separate platter.

4 Cook the shallots and garlic in the oil for about 5 to 7 minutes, until gently browned. Remove them to the platter along with the fennel.

5 Add the vegetable broth, vinegar, and vanilla bean and bring to a gentle simmer. Reduce for about 10 minutes.

6 Season the halibut with salt and pepper. Set it into the poaching liquid and cook for about 4 minutes on one side. Flip and add all of the vegetables to the pan, including the snow peas.

7 Cook for another 4 minutes until the fish flakes easily with a fork and all of the vegetables are heated through. Discard the vanilla bean before serving.

SHRIMP SCAMPI

Serves: 2   **Prep Time:** 5 minutes   **Cook Time:** 15 minutes

Zucchini noodles are a grain-free alternative to traditional pasta, making them easier on your digestive system than either wheat or gluten-free pastas. To make this low-FODMAP, omit the shallots and garlic, and add ¼ cup of thinly sliced green onions.

2 medium zucchini

Sea salt

¼ cup extra-virgin olive oil

1 pound shrimp, peeled and deveined

2 shallots, minced

2 garlic cloves, minced

2 plum tomatoes, seeded and diced

⅛ teaspoon red chile flakes

Zest and juice of 1 lemon

¼ cup chopped fresh flat-leaf parsley

1 Run the zucchini through a spiralizer, or use a vegetable peeler to cut them into long, thin ribbons. Set the noodles in a colander over the sink and sprinkle generously with salt. Allow to sit for 10 minutes, then rinse briefly and squeeze excess moisture from the noodles.

2 Heat the olive oil in a large skillet over medium–high heat. Sauté the shrimp until just cooked through, about 5 to 7 minutes. Remove the cooked shrimp to a clean dish.

3 Return the pan to the stove and lower the heat to medium. Cook the shallots and garlic for 2 minutes, until slightly softened and fragrant. Add the tomatoes, red chile flakes, and lemon zest. Cook for another 2 minutes.

4 Add the zucchini noodles to the pan and cook for 1 to 2 minutes, until just heated through. Return the shrimp to the pan and shower with lemon juice and parsley. Cook for another 1 to 2 minutes and then serve.

SALMON WITH HONEY DIJON BABY BOK CHOY

Serves: 2   **Prep Time:** 5 minutes   **Cook Time:** 5 minutes

Salmon is a rich source of omega-3 fats, which nourish your gut. Choose wild salmon if possible. Farmed salmon contains high amounts of inflammatory omega-6 fats and environmental contaminants due to its confinement and processed diet.

3 tablespoons extra-virgin olive oil, divided

2 skinless salmon fillets, 4 to 6 ounces each

Sea salt

Freshly ground black pepper

Zest and juice of 1 orange

1 tablespoon Dijon mustard

1 tablespoon raw honey

6 to 8 baby bok choy, roughly chopped

2 tablespoons toasted sesame seeds, for serving

1 Heat 2 tablespoons of the oil in a large skillet over medium heat. Season the salmon fillets with salt and pepper. Sear on each side for 2 to 3 minutes, allowing a nice crust to form. The interior should still be a darker shade of pink, but not raw and mushy. Remove the salmon fillets to individual serving plates. They will continue to cook after being removed from the heat.

2 In a medium bowl, whisk together the orange juice and zest, Dijon mustard, and honey.

3 Heat the remaining 1 tablespoon of the oil over medium heat in a large skillet. Stir fry the bok choy for 1 minute, add the orange and honey mixture, and cook until thoroughly wilted.

4 Serve with a sprinkle of sesame seeds alongside the salmon.

STEAMED MUSSELS

Serves: 2   **Prep Time:** 10 minutes   **Cook Time:** 15 minutes

It doesn't get any easier than this recipe for steamed mussels. Make sure to thoroughly scrub and rinse the mussels before using and discard any that are broken or already opened. Serve with Roasted Rosemary Parsnips (page 182).

1 yellow onion, minced

2 garlic cloves, minced

2 thyme sprigs

2 tablespoons extra-virgin olive oil

2 pounds mussels, cleaned and sorted

½ cup dry white wine

1 cup Chicken Bone Broth (page 57)

Sea salt

Freshly ground black pepper

½ cup roughly chopped fresh flat-leaf parsley

1 lemon, cut into wedges, for serving

1 Combine the onion, garlic, thyme, and olive oil in a large pot. Cook over medium heat until the onion begins to soften, about 5 minutes.

2 Add the mussels, white wine, and broth to the pot. Season with salt and pepper and give everything a good toss. Cover and cook for about 10 minutes, until the mussels open.

3 Transfer to a serving dish and garnish with the parsley and lemon wedges.

SHRIMP AND COLLARDS

Serves: 2 to 4   **Prep Time:** 10 minutes   **Cook Time:** 25 minutes

It's often difficult to get enough calories on a grain-free diet. Bacon makes it a little easier and so delicious.

2 slices applewood-smoked bacon, thinly sliced

1 bunch collard greens, ribs removed, cut into thin ribbons

Sea salt

Freshly ground black pepper

1 pound large shrimp, peeled and deveined

1 Cook the bacon in a large skillet over medium–low heat until it is crisp and has rendered most of its fat, about 10 minutes.

2 Transfer the bacon to a separate dish with a slotted spoon. Crumble when cool.

3 Increase the heat to medium, add the collard greens to the pan, and season with salt and pepper. Cook for 10 minutes, until soft but still chewy. Transfer to a serving dish and toss with the bacon.

4 In the same skillet, sear the shrimp until just cooked through, about 5 minutes. Season with salt and pepper and set them on top of the collard greens. Serve immediately.

PROSCIUTTO-WRAPPED SCALLOPS

Serves: 2   **Prep Time:** 10 minutes   **Cook Time:** 6 to 8 minutes

This savory, protein-rich entrée is delicious over a simple bed of mixed greens or with Southwestern Roasted Butternut Squash (page 181).

4 slices prosciutto

8 large sea scallops

Sea salt

Freshly ground black pepper

2 tablespoons extra-virgin olive oil

1 Cut the prosciutto slices in half lengthwise.

2 Pat the scallops dry with a paper towel and wrap 1 strip of prosciutto around the edge of each one. If it will not stick, use a toothpick to secure. Season the scallops lightly with salt and pepper.

3 Heat the olive oil in a large skillet over medium heat. Sear the scallops for about 3 minutes on each side until browned outside and cooked through.

BEEF BOURGUIGNON

Serves: 2 to 4   **Prep Time:** 10 minutes   **Cook Time:** 2½ to 3 hours

I've been cooking beef bourguignon for several years, and this is my absolute favorite rendition of the classic French dish. It is especially nourishing to a sensitive gut because it contains chicken bone broth, which adds body to the luxurious sauce, and it omits wheat flour. The vegetables soften, almost melting into the stew, making them easily digestible. If you are sensitive to FODMAPs, omit or reduce the amount of onions and garlic until you're able to tolerate them.

2 tablespoons rendered bacon fat or coconut oil, divided

1 pound beef chuck, trimmed of all visible fat, cut into 1-inch cubes

Sea salt

Freshly ground black pepper

2 cups halved cremini or button mushrooms

1 yellow onion, halved and sliced in thick half circles

2 garlic cloves, smashed

2 cups dry red wine

3 carrots, peeled, halved, and cut into 3-inch segments

2 fresh thyme sprigs

2 cups Chicken Bone Broth (page 57)

1 Heat 1 tablespoon of the bacon fat in a medium size pot over medium–high heat. Pat the beef dry with paper towels and season on all sides with salt and pepper.

2 Brown the meat in the pan on all sides, about 30 to 45 seconds per side. You may have to do this in batches so as not to crowd the pan. Remove the meat to a separate bowl.

3 Add the remaining tablespoon of bacon fat to the pot and brown the mushrooms for about 2 minutes.

4 Add the onion and garlic and cook for about 30 seconds. Pour in the wine and deglaze the pot, scrapping up all of the delicious browned bits. Return the meat and any accumulated juices to the pot. Add the carrots, thyme, and chicken bone broth. Give everything a stir.

5 Cover and cook over medium-low heat at the barest simmer for 1½ to 2 hours, until the meat is nearly tender. Remove the lid and continue simmering for another 30 minutes, until the sauce is reduced somewhat and the meat is meltingly tender.

BURGER STACKS
WITH CARAMELIZED ONIONS

Serves: 4   **Prep Time:** 10 minutes   **Cook Time:** 25 minutes

Initially, I thought burgers without buns weren't worth the mess. But eventually I came to appreciate that I could taste all of the delicious flavors of the condiments and the juices of the meat when they weren't soaked up by the bun. These can either be wrapped in lettuce leaves or plated and eaten with a fork, as described here.

1 yellow onion, thinly sliced

2 tablespoons extra-virgin olive oil

1 pound ground chuck

¼ cup tomato ketchup, without high-fructose corn syrup

2 tablespoons Dijon mustard

2 tablespoons mayonnaise

2 tomatoes, thinly sliced

1 cup thinly sliced lettuce

Sea salt

Freshly ground black pepper

1 Combine the onion and olive oil in a large skillet over medium-low heat. Season with salt. Cook, stirring often, until the onions are soft and beginning to caramelize, about 15 minutes. Transfer them to a separate dish.

2 Season the ground chuck thoroughly with salt and pepper and form into 4 patties. Raise the temperature to medium and cook them in the same skillet for about 5 minutes on each side, for medium, or until they reach your desired level of doneness. Do not press on the patties with a spatula, which will release all of the juices.

3 Whisk together the ketchup, Dijon mustard, and mayonnaise. Set aside.

4 Allow the burgers to rest for a few minutes before serving. Set each one on an individual plate and top with the dressing, tomatoes, caramelized onions, and lettuce.

BEEF AND GREEN BEAN STIR-FRY

Serves: 4   **Prep Time:** 10 minutes, plus 30 minutes inactive time
Cook Time: 15 minutes

This spicy stir-fry comes together quickly, especially if you make the marinade ahead of time. For low-FODMAP, omit the garlic.

1 teaspoon Chinese five spice powder

1 tablespoon minced fresh ginger

2 garlic cloves, minced

¼ teaspoon red chile flakes

2 tablespoons gluten-free, low-sodium soy sauce

2 tablespoons rice vinegar

1 pound boneless beef top round, thinly sliced on a bias

2 tablespoons sesame oil

1 pound green beans, cut into 2-inch pieces

2 green onions (green parts only) thinly sliced

1 lime, cut into wedges, for serving

1 In a large bowl, combine the Chinese five spice powder, ginger, garlic, red chile flakes, soy sauce, and rice vinegar. Coat the beef in the mixture and set aside to marinate for 30 minutes. Remove the meat from the marinade, shaking off any excess liquid, and pat dry, reserving the leftover marinade.

2 Heat the oil in a large skillet or wok over medium–high heat until almost smoking. Pan-fry the beef until browned and just cooked through, about 5 minutes. Transfer it to a separate dish to rest. Do this in two batches so as not to crowd the pan.

3 Place the green beans in the pan and sauté for 4 to 5 minutes, until al dente.

4 Add the beef and any accumulated juices along with the remaining marinade. Cook for 1 to 2 minutes until the liquid is slightly reduced. Top with green onions and serve with the lime wedges.

STEAK AND VEGETABLE SHISH KEBABS

Serves: 4   **Prep Time:** 5 minutes, plus 30 minutes to 8 hours inactive time   **Cook Time:** 10 minutes

These kebabs are perfect for feeding a crowd. For a low-FODMAP version, omit the onion and mushrooms and use more of the other vegetables.

¼ cup red wine vinegar

2 tablespoons extra-virgin olive oil, divided

1 teaspoon Dijon mustard

1 teaspoon minced fresh rosemary

1 teaspoon sea salt

Freshly ground black pepper

1 pound sirloin steak, cut into 1-inch cubes

1 pint grape tomatoes

8 ounces button mushrooms

1 green bell pepper, cut into 1-inch pieces

1 medium zucchini, cut into 1-inch pieces

1 red onion, cut into 1-inch pieces

1 In a small bowl, whisk together the vinegar, 1 tablespoon of the olive oil, and the mustard, rosemary, salt, and a few grinds of black pepper.

2 Place the steak in a non–reactive dish and coat with the marinade. Allow to marinate for at least 30 minutes or up to 8 hours in the refrigerator.

3 Remove the steak from the marinade and pat dry. Thread the steak onto bamboo skewers along with the tomatoes, mushrooms, bell pepper, zucchini, and onion. Brush the vegetables with the remaining tablespoon of oil.

4 Preheat an outdoor grill or grill pan to medium–high heat. Place the skewers on the grill for 5 minutes, flip and cook for another 5 minutes, or until they reach your desired level of doneness.

14

GUT-HEALING SIDE DISHES

Mashed Parsnips

Cauliflower Rice

Sweet Potato Fries

Zucchini Hummus

Pan-Seared Asparagus

Southwestern Roasted Butternut Squash

Roasted Rosemary Parsnips

Stewed Kale and Dates

Green Beans with Bacon

Eggplant Confit

Oven-Roasted Fennel with Orange

Roasted Pepper Salad

MASHED PARSNIPS

Serves: 2   **Prep Time:** 5 minutes   **Cook Time:** 15 to 20 minutes

Parsnips are a low-FODMAP root vegetable. They resemble thick carrots with a beautiful ivory hue.

4 to 6 parsnips, about 1 pound, peeled and cut into 1-inch pieces

1 cup Chicken Bone Broth (page 57) or low-sodium vegetable broth

1 cup full-fat coconut milk

¼ teaspoon sea salt

1 thyme sprig

2 garlic cloves, smashed

1 Place all of the ingredients in a medium pot. Bring to a simmer over medium–low heat. Cover and cook for 15 to 20 minutes, or until the parsnips are tender.

2 Drain the parsnips, reserving the cooking liquid. Discard the thyme sprig and garlic cloves.

3 Return the parsnips to the pot and mash with a potato masher, adding the cooking liquid as needed to reach the desired consistency.

CAULIFLOWER RICE

Serves: 2   **Prep Time:** 5 minutes   **Cook Time:** 5 minutes

Cauliflower makes a nice stand-in for rice in a grain-free diet. It can be served raw, but it is more easily digestible if you cook it briefly.

1 head cauliflower

1 tablespoon extra-virgin olive oil

Sea salt

Freshly ground black pepper

1 Break the cauliflower into large florets and put them into a food processor fitted with the standard blade. Pulse until it is coarsely chopped and resembles rice.

2 Heat the olive oil in a large skillet over medium heat. Add the cauliflower and sauté for about 5 minutes, until heated through and beginning to soften. Season with salt and pepper and serve.

SWEET POTATO FRIES

Serves: 2 to 4   **Prep Time:** 5 minutes   **Cook Time:** 45 minutes

These basic oven fries are a staple in my house, and I have come to prefer their flavor to that of white-potato fries. Both are rich in nutrients. If you have a particularly sensitive gut, make sure to peel the sweet potatoes before slicing.

4 medium sweet potatoes, scrubbed

2 tablespoons coconut oil, melted

Sea salt

1 Preheat the oven to 400°F.

2 Slice the sweet potatoes into ½–inch–thick spears and spread them out on a rimmed baking sheet. Drizzle with the coconut oil and toss to coat. Season with salt.

3 Bake uncovered for 45 minutes, or until the bottoms are gently browned and they are somewhat shriveled on top.

ZUCCHINI HUMMUS

Yields: 1 cup   **Prep Time:** 5 minutes   **Cook Time:** 0 minutes

If you find chickpeas difficult to digest, you'll love this hummus made from zucchini. To further improve its digestibility, steam the zucchini for 5 minutes before adding it to the blender.

¼ cup lemon juice

2 tablespoons extra-virgin olive oil

¼ cup tahini

2 garlic cloves, minced

1 large zucchini, peeled and diced

Sea salt

Freshly ground black pepper

Combine all of the ingredients in a blender in the order listed and purée until smooth, scraping down the sides as needed. Season with salt and pepper.

PAN-SEARED ASPARAGUS

Serves: 2   **Prep Time:** 5 minutes   **Cook Time:** 5 minutes

For years I trimmed the woody ends of asparagus with a sharp knife. However, the best way to trim them is to snap off the ends using your hands. They snap where the tender portion of the shoot meets the woody portion (though certainly they'll break anywhere they are tender).

1 bunch asparagus, woody ends trimmed

2 tablespoons extra-virgin olive oil

Sea salt

1 tablespoon red wine vinegar

1 Coat the asparagus in the olive oil.

2 Heat a large stainless-steel or cast-iron skillet over high heat until the pan is very hot. Sear the asparagus for about 5 minutes, shaking the pan to ensure they brown on all sides.

3 Remove the asparagus to a serving platter. Toss with a generous pinch of sea salt and the red wine vinegar.

SOUTHWESTERN ROASTED BUTTERNUT SQUASH

Serves: 2   **Prep Time:** 5 minutes   **Cook Time:** 40 to 45 minutes

Butternut squash is a delicious alternative to roasted potatoes. It is both low-FODMAP and allowed on the Specific Carbohydrate Diet.

1 whole butternut squash, peeled, seeded, and cut into 1-inch cubes

2 tablespoons olive oil

1 teaspoon ground cumin

1 teaspoon smoked paprika

1 teaspoon ground coriander

¼ teaspoon cayenne pepper

¼ teaspoon sea salt

Juice of 1 lime

1 Preheat the oven to 375°F.

2 In a large bowl, toss the butternut squash with the olive oil until thoroughly coated. Season with the cumin, smoked paprika, coriander, cayenne, and salt and toss to coat.

3 Spread the squash over a rimmed baking sheet and roast uncovered for 40 to 45 minutes, or until gently browned and tender.

4 Just before serving, drizzle the lime juice over the squash.

ROASTED ROSEMARY PARSNIPS

Serves: 2 to 4   **Prep Time:** 5 minutes   **Cook Time:** 35 to 40 minutes

Oven fries take on a whole new dimension when you use parsnips. They're best in the wintertime when parsnips are in season.

1½ pounds parsnips, peeled

2 tablespoons extra-virgin olive oil

1 tablespoon minced fresh rosemary

Sea salt

Freshly ground pepper

1 Preheat the oven to 375°F.

2 Cut the parsnips into ½-inch-thick spears. Spread them out on a rimmed baking sheet. Drizzle with the olive oil and rosemary and toss to coat thoroughly. Season with salt and pepper.

3 Roast uncovered for 35 to 40 minutes, until browned and beginning to caramelize. Serve immediately.

STEWED KALE AND DATES

Serves: 2   **Prep Time:** 5 minutes   **Cook Time:** 25 minutes

This sweet and savory side dish goes well with Prosciutto-Wrapped Scallops (page 169) or Basic Roasted Chicken (page 152).

2 tablespoons olive oil

1 small yellow onion, halved and thinly sliced

Sea salt

4 Medjool dates, pitted and thinly sliced

1 large bunch Lacinato kale

½ cup Chicken Bone Broth (page 57)

2 teaspoons red wine vinegar

Freshly ground black pepper

1 Heat the olive oil in a large skillet over medium–low heat. Cook the onion with a generous pinch of sea salt for about 5 minutes, until it begins to soften. Add the dates to the pan and cook for another 5 minutes.

2 Remove the ribs from the kale leaves. Chop the leaves into 2-inch pieces and finely dice the ribs. Add the kale to the pan along with the chicken broth, vinegar, and a few grinds of black pepper.

3 Cook for 10 to 15 minutes, until the kale is very soft and nearly all of the liquid has evaporated.

GREEN BEANS WITH BACON

Serves: 2   **Prep Time:** 5 minutes   **Cook Time:** 25 minutes

The best green beans I have ever had are first blanched and shocked and then given a very brief pan sear. This technique yields a tender vegetable with a crisp snap. However, if you're short on time, feel free to skip that step and sauté the green beans for slightly longer in the final step.

1 pound green beans, stems removed

2 slices applewood-smoked bacon, thinly sliced

2 shallots, minced

1 teaspoon apple cider vinegar

Sea salt

Freshly ground black pepper

1 Bring a large pot of salted water to a boil. Also prepare a large bowl full of ice water. Plunge the green beans into the boiling water and cook for 2 to 3 minutes until bright green. Immediately transfer them with tongs or a slotted spoon to the ice-water bath to cool. Drain and keep cool. This step may be done ahead of time.

2 In a large skillet over medium-low heat, cook the bacon pieces until most of the fat is rendered, about 10 minutes. Transfer them to a separate dish.

3 Cook the shallots in the bacon fat until soft, about 5 to 7 minutes. Transfer them to the dish with the bacon.

4 Increase the heat to medium-high. Sauté the green beans in the remaining bacon fat until they are just heated through, about 2 minutes. Add the bacon and shallots back to the pan along with the vinegar, and give everything a good toss. Season with salt and pepper.

EGGPLANT CONFIT

Serves: 2   **Prep Time:** 5 minutes   **Cook Time:** 45 to 50 minutes

I love using the word "confit" (cone-FEE) because it adds instant elegance to a recipe. But the truth is, it just means cooking food in fat, usually its own. It's one of my favorite ways to cook eggplant, because the vegetable acts like a sponge and soaks up all of the olive oil while melting into an easily digestible, tender, creamy texture.

1 medium eggplant	Sea salt
2 shallots, minced	Freshly ground black pepper
2 tablespoons roughly chopped fresh mint	⅓ cup olive oil
	Balsamic vinegar, for serving

1 Preheat the oven to 325°F.

2 Slice the eggplant horizontally into ½-inch-thick rounds. Combine it in a large mixing bowl with the shallots and mint. Season with salt and pepper. Add the olive oil and toss to coat thoroughly.

3 Spread the eggplant onto a rimmed baking sheet. Bake uncovered for 45 to 50 minutes, or until the eggplant is caramelized on the bottom and very tender. Sprinkle with balsamic vinegar just before serving.

OVEN-ROASTED FENNEL WITH ORANGE

Serves: 2   **Prep Time:** 5 minutes   **Cook Time:** 45 minutes

Fennel bulb and orange are a match made in heaven. I'm sure you'll agree when you try this succulent roasted vegetable.

2 fennel bulbs, trimmed and cut into 8 wedges each

¼ cup extra-virgin olive oil

Zest and juice of 2 oranges

¼ teaspoon red chile flakes

Sea salt

Freshly ground black pepper

1 tablespoon red wine vinegar

1 Preheat the oven to 375°F.

2 Spread the fennel out onto a rimmed baking sheet. Drizzle with the olive oil and season with the orange zest, red chile flakes, and salt and pepper. Toss gently to coat.

3 Roast uncovered for 35 minutes, or until the fennel is tender and beginning to brown.

4 While the fennel is roasting, combine the orange juice and vinegar. Pour this over the fennel and give everything a good toss. Return to the oven for another 10 minutes.

ROASTED PEPPER SALAD

Serves: 2   **Prep Time:** 5 minutes   **Cook Time:** 4 minutes, plus 10 minutes inactive time

Choose red, yellow, and orange sweet bell peppers for a pretty colored salad. This is delicious served with grilled steak and can easily be prepared over a grill instead of under a broiler.

4 sweet bell peppers, cored and halved

2 tablespoons extra-virgin olive oil

Sea salt

Freshly ground black pepper

1 teaspoon cumin seeds

½ teaspoon smoked paprika

1 garlic clove, minced

Zest and juice of 1 lemon

1 Preheat the broiler to high. Place the oven rack on the top level, so the peppers will be about 2 inches from the heating element.

2 Place the peppers skin-side up on a broiler pan. Coat the skin lightly with some of the olive oil. Place them under the broiler for 3 to 4 minutes, or until charred. Carefully transfer the peppers to a separate dish, season with salt and pepper, and cover tightly with a lid or foil.

3 Allow the peppers to steam for about 10 minutes.

4 Meanwhile, combine the cumin seeds, paprika, garlic, lemon zest and juice, and remaining olive oil in a small serving bowl.

5 Remove the charred skin from the peppers and slice the flesh into long, thin strips. Place them in the serving bowl and toss gently to coat. Serve warm or at room temperature.

APPENDIX

GLOSSARY OF TERMS

Autoimmune disease: a disease in which the immune system attacks healthy tissues or organs in the human body. A few examples of autoimmune diseases include type 1 diabetes, celiac disease, rheumatoid arthritis, and multiple sclerosis.

Dysbiosis: microbial imbalance in the gastrointestinal tract; either an overgrowth of pathological organisms, limited total microbial population, lack of diversity, or movement of bacteria from the colon into the small intestine.

Enterocytes: cells lining the intestines that absorb nutrients and secrete mucus.

FODMAPs: fermentable carbohydrates, including oligosaccharides, disaccharides, monosaccharides, and polyols, that facilitate a healthy microbiome in most people but can cause digestive discomfort in some, particularly when consumed in excess. A low-FODMAP diet is often recommended for a period of time for those with irritable bowel syndrome.

Inflammation: A healthy physical response to injury or toxic substances that removes harmful tissues or substances and initiates healing. Chronic inflammation may damage surrounding tissues and contribute to disease.

Intestinal permeability: the weakening of junctures between enterocytes in the intestines, allowing foreign substances to escape the intestinal lumen (tube) and enter the bloodstream. Also known as leaky gut.

Microbiome: the genes present in the organisms that comprise the microbiota.

Microbiota: the trillions of bacteria, viruses, and fungi inhabiting your gastrointestinal tract.

Prebiotic: foods containing a type of fiber that passes through the gastrointestinal tract undigested and stimulates the growth of healthy bacteria in the colon.

Probiotic: foods containing live, active bacterial cultures that bolster the population of healthy bacteria in the gastrointestinal tract.

Saccharide: carbohydrates, including sugar, starch, and cellulose. Saccharides vary in chemical structure and include mono-, di-, oligo-, and polysaccharide forms.

Short-chain fatty acids: microbes produced by the gut during fermentation in the colon. Butyrate is one short-chain fatty acid that is a source of energy for the colon and has anti-inflammatory and anticancer properties.

REFERENCES

The American Gut. Accessed September 2015.
http://americangut.org.

Arranga, Teri, Viadro, Claire, and Underwood, Lauren. *Bugs, Bowels, and Behavior: The Groundbreaking Story of the Gut-Brain Connection.* New York: Skyhorse Publishing, 2013.

Azvolinsky, Anna. "Sugar Substitutes, Gut Bacteria, and Glucose Intolerance." The Scientist. September 17, 2014. Accessed November 6, 2015. http://www.the-scientist.com/?articles.view/articleNo/41033/title/Sugar-Substitutes—Gut-Bacteria—and-Glucose-Intolerance.

Ballantyne, Sarah. "Is It Paleo? Guar Gum, Xanthan Gum, and Lecithin, Oh My!" The Paleo Mom. December 4, 2014. Accessed November 8, 2015. http://www.thepaleomom.com/2014/12/is-it-paleo-guar-gum-xanthan-gum-and-lecithin-oh-my.html.

Biedermann L., et al. "Smoking Cessation Induces Profound Changes in the Composition of the Intestinal Microbiota in Humans." *PLoS One* 8, no. 3 (March 14, 2013). http://journals.plos.org/plosone/article?id=10.1371/journal.pone.0059260.

Cowan, M. M., "Plant Products as Antimicrobial Agents." *Clinical Microbiology Reviews* (October 12, 1999). http://www.ncbi.nlm.nih.gov/pmc/articles/PMC88925.

DiBaise J. K., et al. "Impact of the Gut Microbiota on the Development of Obesity: Current Concepts." *American Journal of Gastroenterology Supplements* 1 (2012): 22–27. http://www.nature.com/ajgsup/journal/v1/n1/full/ajgsup20125a.html.

Evolutionary Medicine. "Which Fats Are Good for You and Your Microbiota?" December 31, 2014. Accessed November 9, 2015. http://evolutionmedicine.com/2014/12/31/recent-articles-on-fat-and-microbiota.

Guyenet, Stephan. "Butyric Acid: an Ancient Controller of Metabolism, Inflammation and Stress Resistance?" Whole Health Source Nutrition and Science. December 7, 2009. Accessed November 2, 2015. http://wholehealthsource.blogspot. com/2009/12/butyric-acid-ancient-controller-of.html.

Heritage Integrative Healthcare. "The Importance of Chewing your Food." Accessed November 5, 2015. http://heritageihc.com/blog/ chewing-your-food.

Knowlton, Andrew. "Do Jerusalem Artichokes Cause Diarrhea?" *Bon Appétit.* February 13, 2009. Accessed November 9, 2015. http:// www.bonappetit.com/columns/the-foodist/article/do-jerusalem-artichokes-cause-diarrhea.

Konturek P. C., Brzozowski, T., and Konturek, S. J. "Stress and the Gut: Pathophysiology, Clinical Consequences, Diagnostic Approach, and Treatment Options." *Journal of Physiology and Pharmacology* 2, no. 6 (2011): 591–99. http://www.jpp.krakow.pl/journal/ archive/12_11/pdf/591_12_11_article.pdf.

Kresser, Chris. "9 Steps to Perfect Health—#5 Heal Your Gut." February 24, 2011. Accessed September 2015. http://chriskresser. com/9-steps-to-perfect-health-5-heal-your-gut.

Kresser, Chris. "A Healthy Gut Is the Hidden Key to Weight Loss." October 29, 2010. Accessed November 11, 2015. http://chriskresser. com/a-healthy-gut-is-the-hidden-key-to-weight-loss.

Kresser, Chris. "How Resistant Starch Will Help to Make You Healthier and Thinner." August 14, 2014. Accessed November 11, 2015. http://chriskresser.com/how-resistant-starch-will-help-to-make-you-healthier-and-thinner.

Kresser, Chris. "RHR: How to Restore Healthy Gut Flora over the Long Term." June 25, 2014. Accessed November 6, 2015. http:// chriskresser.com/how-to-restore-healthy-gut-flora-over-the-long-term.

Liu, Z., et al. "Prebiotic Effects of Almonds and Almond Skins on Intestinal Microbiota in Healthy Adult Humans." *Anaerobe* 26 (April 2014): 1–6. http://www.ncbi.nlm.nih.gov/pubmed/24315808.

Martin, Francois-Pierre J., et al. "Metabolic Effects of Dark Chocolate Consumption on Energy, Gut Microbiota, and Stress-Related Metabolism in Free-Living Subjects." *Journal of Proteome Research* (October 2009). http://www.researchgate.net/profile/Francois-Pierre_Martin/publication/26877619_Metabolic_Effects_of_Dark_Chocolate_Consumption_on_Energy_Gut_Microbiota_and_Stress-Related_Metabolism_in_Free-Living_Subjects/links/09e4151025f8d44fac000000.pdf.

Mercola, Joseph. "'Good Gut Bacteria' May Help Fight Obesity." Mercola.com. June 8, 2011. Accessed November 8, 2015. http://articles.mercola.com/sites/articles/archive/2011/06/18/good-gut-bacteria-may-help-fight-obesity.aspx.

Mercola, Joseph. "Processed Foods Hurt Your Immune System and Gut Health." Mercola.com. July 16, 2014. Accessed October 2015. http://articles.mercola.com/sites/articles/archive/2014/07/16/processed-foods-immune-system-gut-health.aspx.

Montenegro, L., et al. "Non-Steroidal Anti-Inflammatory Drug Induced Damage on Lower Gastro-Intestinal Tract: Is There an Involvement of Microbiota?" *Current Drug Safety* 9, no. 3, (2014): 196–204. http://www.ncbi.nlm.nih.gov/pubmed/24809527.

Ritz, B. "Red Wine Polyphenols' Effects on Gut Microbiota Ecology; Reduction of Clostridium in the Human Gut Could Offer Promise for a Range of Conditions." *Natural Medicine Journal* 4, no. 8 (August 2012). http://www.naturalmedicinejournal.com/journal/2012-08/red-wine-polyphenols-effects-gut-microbiota-ecology.

Rubin, Jordan S. "How to Restore Digestive Health." Weston Price Foundation. September 22, 2004. Accessed September 2015. http://www.westonaprice.org/modern-diseases/how-to-restore-digestive-health.

Samsel, A., and Seneff, S. "Glyphosate's Suppression of Cytochrome P450 Enzymes and Amino Acid Biosynthesis by the Gut Microbiome: Pathways to Modern Diseases." *Entropy* 15, no. 4 (2013): 1416–63. http://www.mdpi.com/1099-4300/15/4/1416.

Sisson, Mark. "16 Things that Affect Your Gut Bacteria." Mark's Daily Apple. Accessed November 6, 2015. http://www.marksdailyapple.com/16-things-that-affect-your-gut-bacteria/#axzz3qjUydA8s.

Spreadbury, I. "Comparison with Ancestral Diets Suggests Dense Acellular Carbohydrates Promote an Inflammatory Microbiota, and May Be the Primary Dietary Cause of Leptin Resistance and Obesity." *Dove Press* no. 5 (July 6, 2012): 175–89. https://www.dovepress.com/comparison-with-ancestral-diets-suggests-dense-acellular-carbohydrates-peer-reviewed-article-DMSO-MVP.

Turnbaugh, P., et al. "The Effect of Diet on the Human Gut Microbiome: A Metagenomic Analysis in Humanized Gnotobiotic Mice." *Science Translational Medicine* 1, no. 6 (November 11, 2009). http://stm.sciencemag.org/content/1/6/6ra14.full.

Ukhanova, M., et al. "Effects of Almond and Pistachio Consumption on Gut Microbiota Composition in a Randomised Cross-Over Human Feeding Study." *British Journal of Nutrition* 111, no. 12 (June 28, 2014): 2146–52. http://www.ncbi.nlm.nih.gov/pubmed/24642201.

CONVERSION CHARTS

VOLUME CONVERSIONS

U.S.	U.S. Equivalent	Metric
1 tablespoon (3 teaspoons)	½ fluid ounce	15 milliliters
¼ cup	2 fluid ounces	60 milliliters
⅓ cup	3 fluid ounces	90 milliliters
½ cup	4 fluid ounces	120 milliliters
⅔ cup	5 fluid ounces	150 milliliters
¾ cup	6 fluid ounces	180 milliliters
1 cup	8 fluid ounces	240 milliliters
2 cups	16 fluid ounces	480 milliliters

WEIGHT CONVERSIONS

U.S.	Metric
½ ounce	15 grams
1 ounce	30 grams
2 ounces	60 grams
¼ pound	115 grams
⅓ pound	150 grams
½ pound	225 grams
¾ pound	350 grams
1 pound	450 grams

TEMPERATURE CONVERSIONS

Fahrenheit (°F)	Celsius (°C)
70°F	20°C
100°F	40°C
120°F	50°C
130°F	55°C
140°F	60°C
150°F	65°C
160°F	70°C
170°F	75°C
180°F	80°C
190°F	90°C
200°F	95°C
220°F	105°C
240°F	115°C
260°F	125°C
280°F	140°C
300°F	150°C
325°F	165°C
350°F	175°C
375°F	190°C
400°F	200°C
425°F	220°C
450°F	230°C

RECIPE INDEX

ACKNOWLEDGMENTS

I am so grateful for the amazing publishing team at Ulysses Press, especially Alice, Casie, Keith, Renee, and Kourtney. You guys have been so patient and helped me develop and promote the best possible manuscript every time!

Thank you, Savannah, for giving me my first SCOBY and teaching me how to brew kombucha.

Special thanks to my husband, Rich, for his patience and lending his palate to help me test recipes.

ABOUT THE AUTHOR

Pamela Ellgen is a food blogger, certified personal trainer, and author of several books on cooking, nutrition, and fitness, including *Sheet Pan Paleo*, *Soup & Comfort*, and the bestselling *Healthy Slow Cooker Cookbook*. Her work has been published in *Huffington Post*, LIVESTRONG, *Darling Magazine*, and Spinning.com. She lives in California with her husband and two sons. When she's not in the kitchen, she enjoys surfing and exploring the local farmer's market.